KU-281-991

Contents

· ·

WITHDRAWN FROM STOCK

Introduction

If you want to look and feel great, have more energy and make positive changes to improve your health, this is the book for you.

Over 125,000 people have now tried and tested *BBC Good Food*'s delicious and nutritious Healthy Diet Plans, and they seem to love them as much as we do! Rigorously tested and nutritionally analysed, we believe we've found the perfect formula to boost health and well-being in the tastiest way possible.

Eat the right foods and you will feel re-energised, and you may even see some welcome weight loss – especially if you exercise a little more too, but don't expect to go hungry, this book is packed with healthy recipes created by *BBC Good Food*, so you are safe in the knowledge that they will be delicious and easy to cook too.

The book is divided into 3 different 7-day diet plans, with additional sections on healthy snacks and desserts. Following a plan helps prevent impulsive, unhealthy food choices and keeps you on track to meet your health goals, while each recipe aims to make the most of food in its natural and purest form, a philosophy Kerry Torrens, *Good Food*'s nutritional therapist, will explain over the next few pages.

So what are the benefits of eating like this? Glowing skin, a flatter stomach and heaps of energy, plus you should sleep better and think more clearly. Who wouldn't want that? And if you continue to eat this way beyond the 7 days, you'll also improve your heart health and digestion, and help to balance your hormones.

Each plan has a different focus, whether you want to boost your immune system, eat vegetarian, which can help you to reduce your cholesterol, or flood your body with feel-good nutrients to improve your looks. Once you've completed your chosen 7-day plan, you'll find lots of additional recipes to add variety as you develop your new way of cooking and eating.

Every recipe in the book has a colour photo and has been analysed on a per-serving basis, so you can see exactly what each dish contains – from the calories, fat and sugar right down to the salt quantities. Then we have devised a handy weekly chart incorporating breakfast, lunch and dinner to make the diet easy to follow day-by-day, ensuring that you will get all the nutrition you need. Each day contributes to more than 5 of your 5 a day, keeps within recommended Reference Intakes (RI) for fats, sugar, salt and kcals and follow healthy diet principles.

As you browse through the book look out for the highlighted healthy benefits too, as we will let you know if a recipe is rich in vitamin C, is high in fibre or has 1 or more of your 5 a day.

The recipes mostly cater for two portions; dishes that serve more are suitable for freezing or storing in the fridge for a few days, or are meals or desserts suitable for entertaining.

So if you, like many, are confused about what constitutes a healthy, balanced diet – simply select your preferred plan, and get cooking.

If you love food, eating in a healthy and balanced way has never been easier or more delicious.

Sara

Sara Buenfeld

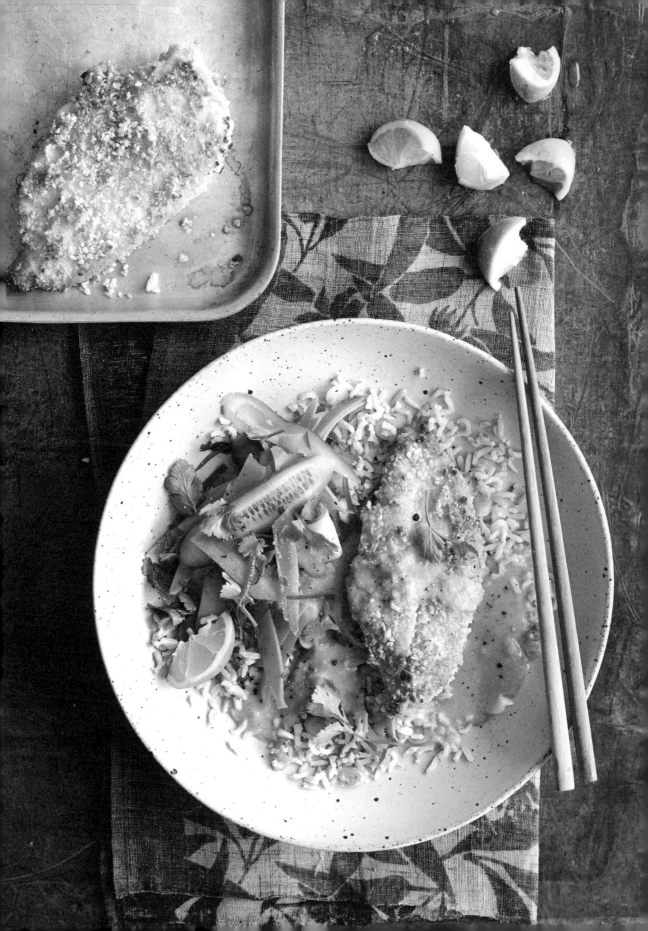

A new way to cook

The key to eating healthily is to avoid processed, refined foods and focus on healthy, natural fats, lean sources of protein and slow-release carbs. We've used foods in their most natural, unprocessed form so you benefit from optimal nourishment. You'll see that all our plans are balanced and include ingredients from all the major food groups. The recipes are easy to prepare and cook and won't demand huge amounts of your time. Here are some simple guidelines to help get you started.

---

10 fruit & veg most likely to contain pesticides*

- ☐ Apples
- ☐ Carrots
- ☐ Celery
- ☐ Grapes
- ☐ Greens, including spinach and kale
- ☐ Peaches and nectarines
- ☐ Peppers
- ☐ Potatoes
- ☐ Strawberries
- ☐ Cherry tomatoes

*correct at time of publication

FOODS TO SHOP FOR

All fresh and frozen fruit and veg
Be mindful of pesticides (see the box below for the fruit and veg likely to contain the most). If buying canned, choose those in water only rather than with added salt or sugar. Opt for unwaxed citrus fruits – if that's not possible, scrub under the tap before using the zest. Coconut and dried fruit are great for enhancing flavour, but avoid those that have been sweetened or preserved with sulphur dioxide.

Lean, unprocessed meat and organic or free-range poultry
Choose the best you can afford – whether that's organic, grass-fed, free-range or simply a leaner cut. Meat is one of those ingredients where the quality really does make a difference to the taste, texture and nutrition of your finished dish. When buying poultry buy the whole bird, when practical, so you can use the carcass for a home-made stock or bone broth.

Fish & seafood
Be mindful of source and variety. Opt for wild rather than farmed fish as they have a superior fat composition. Aim to eat oily fish, that's salmon, trout, sardines or mackerel, at least once a week.

Organic dairy

Where budget permits opt for organic dairy products as these are likely to have a better fat composition with more of the healthy omega-3 variety and are less likely to contain hormones and antibiotics. We've used semi-skimmed or whole milk in our recipes – the fat in milk helps us absorb important fat-soluble vitamins like A and E. Alternatively, try dairy-free alternatives made from scratch, such as oat milk (see box below).

How to make oat & nut milks

Put 100g/4oz oats or 150g/4½oz whole almonds or cashews in a large bowl and cover with water. Leave to soak, preferably overnight or for at least 4 hours if you are short of time.

The next day, drain and tip the oats or nuts into a blender with 750ml/1.3 pints cold water and whizz until smooth.

Pour the mixture into a nut milk bag or a muslin-lined sieve set over a jug, and allow to drip through. Stir the mixture gently with a spoon to speed it up, if you like.

When most of the liquid has filtered into the jug, gather the sides of the bag or muslin together and squeeze tightly with both hands to extract the last of the milk. It will keep in the fridge for a few days.

Grains and pseudo-grains

Go for ones with minimal processing so they remain in their nutritious, whole-grain form. Good options include quinoa, amaranth, millet, buckwheat, freekeh, wholegrain barley and brown/black/wild/red rice. These can be enjoyed as savoury or sweet dishes, for example a tabbouleh like our Barley couscous & prawn tabbouleh on page 108 or as a porridge like our Coconut quinoa & chia porridge on page 92.

Beans and pulses

We have used canned beans in many of our recipes for convenience. If using dried you can make them more digestible by soaking (or activating) them in water overnight before cooking, then using in the recipes.

Nuts and seeds

Choose unsalted ones, including their oils and butters. If you are buying nut butters, again, avoid added salt as well as sugar and palm oil. Instead why not make your own? Try our Cashew spread on page 238 and Almond butter page 240. Nut milks are increasingly popular, but many shop-bought versions have emulsifiers and stabilisers and often very little nut content! Try making your own and you'll definitely taste the difference – see box left.

Opt for a range of seeds including pumpkin, flaxseed, hemp, sesame and chia – these can be used in dishes or as a finishing flourish to a salad or soup.

Oils for cooking, spreading and dressing

Don't be afraid to include some fat – it is essential to good health. Rapeseed oil has a high smoke point, which means it is a good oil to cook with. It has just 7% saturated fat and makes a useful contribution of heart-friendly omega-3 fatty acids. Other oils to include are cold-pressed olive and nut oils for dressings and drizzles and virgin coconut oil, which has great immune-boosting benefits and because it is a saturate it can be used for cooking at high temperatures. Don't forget butter – nothing works better scraped on hot toast! Butter is a good source of butyric acid, a gut-friendly type of fatty acid – just make sure you buy a brand that is 100% butter and not a plant oil and butter spread.

Vinegars
Balsamic and organic apple cider vinegar are fabulous flavour enhancers. Buy the best you can afford and avoid those processed with sulphur dioxide or with additives like colouring agents.

Herbs and spices
All spices and fresh or dried herbs are useful for enhancing flavour. Some herbs and spices are especially good for our health – turmeric aids digestion and is anti-inflammatory (check out our Turmeric bowl on page 28). We've added little in the way of salt to our recipes, preferring to use naturally salty ingredients like seafood or using herbs, spices and citrus juices to bring out the natural flavours. If you do like to add seasonings, opt for an unrefined salt like Himalayan salt or rock salt rather than regular table salt.

Free-range or organic eggs.
Many people shy away from including eggs on a regular basis, but the latest scientific evidence suggests that eating them as part of a healthy, balanced diet is beneficial for most of us. Eggs are a valuable source of vitamin D, as well as B vitamins and trace minerals, which are important for a healthy nervous system.

FOODS TO AVOID

Refined grains
These are highly processed, so they have a finer texture and longer shelf life, but they are nutritionally inferior. Avoid these white grains and products using them, like cakes, ready-made pastry, shop-bought bread, plus white pasta, couscous and rice.

Refined sugar
Including sugar substitutes that are processed, such as stevia, agave and commercial honey. These are largely empty calories, supplying a sweet hit and nothing more. Including too many sweet foods only encourages a sweet tooth.

Packaged or processed meat and fish
This includes bacon, preserved pork products like Parma ham, sausages, salami, chorizo, as well as smoked fish.

Some shop-bought condiments and dressings
Mayonnaise, ketchup, relish, chutney and mustards are highly processed and contain additives. Ideally make your own. Also avoid commerical packet stock cubes and instead opt for a reduced-salt vegetable bouillon. You'll notice that we use wheat-free tamari instead of soy sauce in our recipes. This is because commercial soy sauce may contain additives such as caramel colouring as well as flavour enhancers.

Anything packaged or processed
Including Quorn and soya meat replacements. Our plans use ingredients in their natural, unprocessed, unrefined form – simply put, they are foods you can recognise.

How to use each plan

We suggest eating the meals as set out in each plan to get the best results. However, if you want to swap or repeat days, or try recipes in other plans, you'll still reap all the benefits of eating whole, unprocessed foods.

Each day supplies under 1,500 kcals and delivers more than 5 of your 5 a day. As a result, with each plan you can expect to cut back on added sugar, lose excess pounds and increase your energy. As our recipes are packed with cleansing fibre, you may initially experience some minor bloating as your system adjusts. This will soon pass and your digestion will feel the better for it.

If you're looking to lose weight, the daily 1,500-kcal intake should be ideal to help you reach your goals. However, if you're particularly active, or you are not interested in weight loss, we have a chapter on healthy snacks that you can eat between meals.

Be sure to devote the time to your meals they deserve, after all eating is one of the pleasures in life – eating slowly and mindfully will help your body register that food is on the way and prevent you from overeating. Research has shown that eating mindfully improves digestion, regulates appetite and helps us enjoy and savour our food. When you first cut down on sugars and caffeine, you may experience a few headaches. Maintain your hydration levels and stick with it and you'll find they soon pass, and you'll feel all the benefits.

Think about these portion sizes

Choose a plate that holds the amount of food you can fit into your cupped hands. This is your portion size for a main meal. Next, divide the plate into quarters – fill one with protein, the second with healthy low-GI carbs and the other two with vegetables and salad.

Here's what a portion should look like:

Protein (poultry, lean meat, eggs, fish, dairy and veggie alternatives like tofu) – the size of the palm of your hand; for cheese the equivalent of two of your fingers

Carbs (brown rice, pasta, bread and potatoes) – about the size of your clenched fist

Fat (butter/spreads) – the size of your thumbnail

WHAT TO DRINK

Herbal teas and filtered water are your best options. If you can't kick the caffeine, one cup of coffee or black or green tea a day isn't the end of the world, but avoid decaffeinated versions as most are processed with chemicals. We suggest avoiding alcohol while doing the plans.

HOW TO SNACK

Try leftover fruit and veg to minimise waste and save money. Nuts and seeds are good choices, or see our suggestions starting on page 226.

Nutrition notes

All the recipes in this book are analysed on their listed ingredients only, excluding optional extras such as serving suggestions or seasoning – and so these quantities are not included. If you serve the portion sizes suggested, you can work out how each recipe fits into your day-to-day diet by comparing the figures with the Reference Intake (RI). These are the recommended daily figures based on an average-sized woman doing an average amount of activity. RIs are not intended as targets, as energy and nutrient requirements vary, but they provide a useful guide as to the amount of energy (kilocalories), fat, saturated fat, carbohydrate, sugar, protein and salt an average woman should consume each day.

Reference Intake (RI)
The figures below for fat, saturated fat, sugar and salt are maximum daily amounts and so should not be exceeded.

Energy (Kilocalories): 2,000
Protein: 50g
Carbohydrate: 260g
Sugar: 90g
Fat: 70g
Saturated fat: 20g
Salt: 6g

Notes & conversion tables

NOTES ON THE RECIPES
- Eggs are large in the UK and Australia and extra large in America unless stated.
- Wash fresh produce before preparation.
- Recipes contain nutritional analyses for 'sugars', which means the total sugar content, including all natural sugars in ingredients, unless otherwise stated.

APPROXIMATE WEIGHT CONVERSIONS
- All the recipes in this book list both metric and imperial measurements. Conversions are approximate and have been rounded up or down. Follow one set of measurements only; do not mix the two.
- Cup measurements, which are used in Australia and America, have not been listed here as they vary from ingredient to ingredient. Kitchen scales should be used to measure dry/solid ingredients.

Good Food is concerned about sustainable sourcing and animal welfare. Where possible, humanely reared meats, sustainably caught fish (see fishonline.org for further information from the Marine Conservation Society) and free-range chickens and eggs are used when recipes are originally tested.

OVEN TEMPERATURES

GAS	°C	°C FAN	°F	OVEN TEMP.
¼	110	90	225	Very cool
½	120	100	250	Very cool
1	140	120	275	Cool or slow
2	150	130	300	Cool or slow
3	160	140	325	Warm
4	180	160	350	Moderate
5	190	170	375	Moderately hot
6	200	180	400	Fairly hot
7	220	200	425	Hot
8	230	210	450	Very hot
9	240	220	475	Very hot

SPOON MEASURES
Spoon measurements are level unless otherwise specified.
- 1 teaspoon (tsp) = 5ml
- 1 tablespoon (tbsp) = 15ml
- 1 Australian tablespoon = 20ml
(Cooks in Australia should measure 3 teaspoons where 1 tablespoon is specified in a recipe)

APPROXIMATE LIQUID CONVERSIONS

Metric	Imperial	AUS	US
50ml	2fl oz	¼ cup	¼ cup
125ml	4fl oz	½ cup	½ cup
175ml	6fl oz	¾ cup	¾ cup
225ml	8fl oz	1 cup	1 cup
300ml	10fl oz/½ pint	½ pint	1¼ cups
450ml	16fl oz	2 cups	2 cups/1 pint
600ml	20fl oz/1 pint	1 pint	2½ cups
1 litre	35fl oz/1¾ pints	1¾ pints	1 quart

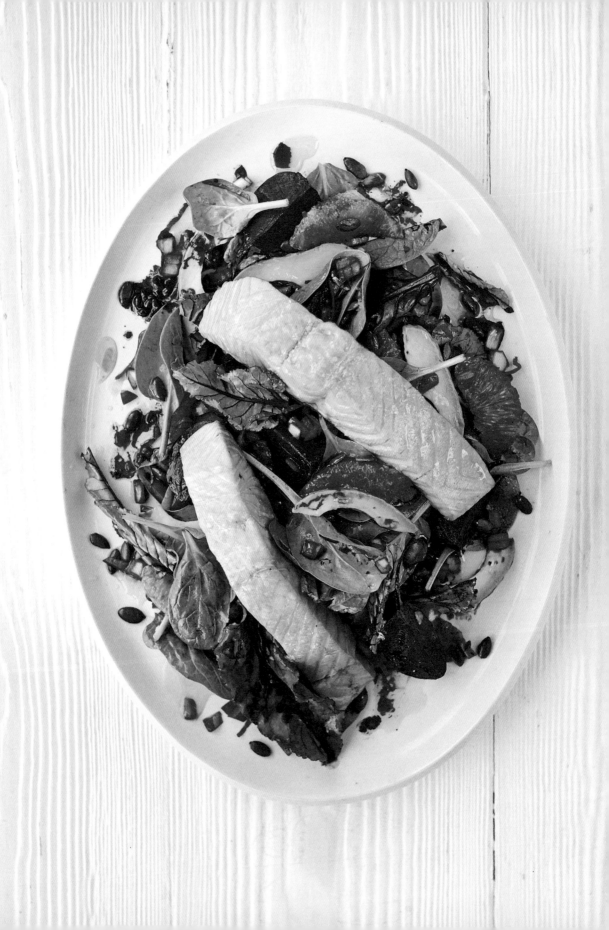

Chapter 1:

THE 7-DAY HEALTH OVERHAUL PLAN

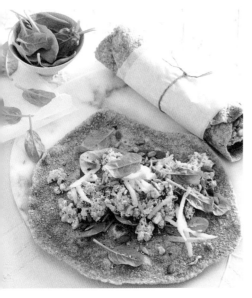

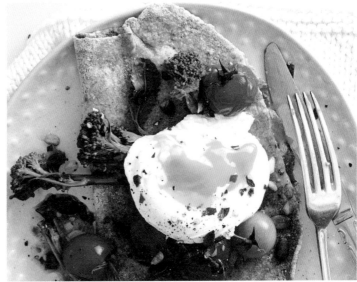

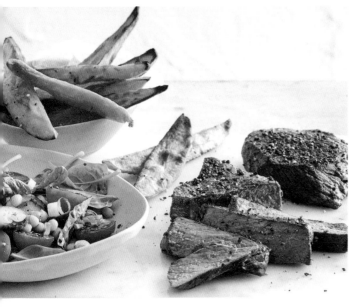

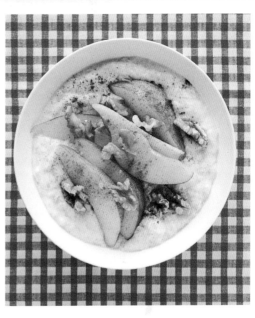

Boost digestion and immunity in 7 days

If you or one of your family tends to suffer one cold after another then you may need to take a closer look at your diet and lifestyle. It's estimated that 60-70% of our immune defences are located in our gut – so what we eat and how we look after our digestive system is key. Stress and burning the candle at both ends, combined with a diet of processed, 'on the hoof' meals will also play its part in making us feel run down.

This 7-day immune support plan is based on natural, unprocessed foods, with meals cooked from scratch, so you get to enjoy them at their most nourishing. Our recipes are based on ingredients with specific properties that support the functioning of the immune system and the health of your gut.

Gut instinct

Throughout our plan we've included naturally fermented or probiotic yogurt. This is a fabulous source of gut-friendly beneficial bacteria. Keeping with our natural philosophy, we've avoided yogurt with added flavours, thickeners and sweeteners in preference for a good quality plain, live whole fat yogurt.

Eating fermented foods regularly helps top up our good gut bacteria and promotes the right environment for these beneficial bacteria to thrive. These gut microbes are important because when attacked by a virus, our gut bacteria leap into action to stop the virus from multiplying and neutralise any toxins it makes. Other fermented foods include kefir, miso, kimchi and sauerkraut, which you can add to complement the plan and boost your intake of beneficial bacteria further if you like.

As well as boosting levels of gut bacteria, it's also important to supply the fuel for them to thrive. These bacteria-friendly foods, typically fibres like inulin, are known as prebiotics and can be found in certain vegetables and fruit like onions and garlic, asparagus and bananas as well as oats. Including these foods regularly helps support the gut environment and strengthen your immune defences. That's why we've included fibre-rich ingredients like chickpeas, beans, lentils, brown rice, nuts, seeds, fruit and veg in our immune-friendly recipes.

Vital vitamins

We all know vitamin C plays a big part in protecting us from coughs and colds, but it's also important in the healing process. Don't limit yourself to citrus fruits – peppers, broccoli and kale are all excellent sources. Vitamin C is light and heat sensitive so use the freshest ingredients or opt for frozen, because these are picked and packed promptly to lock in their vitamin C goodness. Vitamin C is lost during the cooking process, so follow our recipes to minimise cooking time. Also, because vitamin C is water-soluble, when you are cooking vegetables as an extra side dish be sure to make use of the cooking liquor, say in a sauce or stock or adding to soups or stews. Alternatively, steam or lightly stir-fry your vegetables.

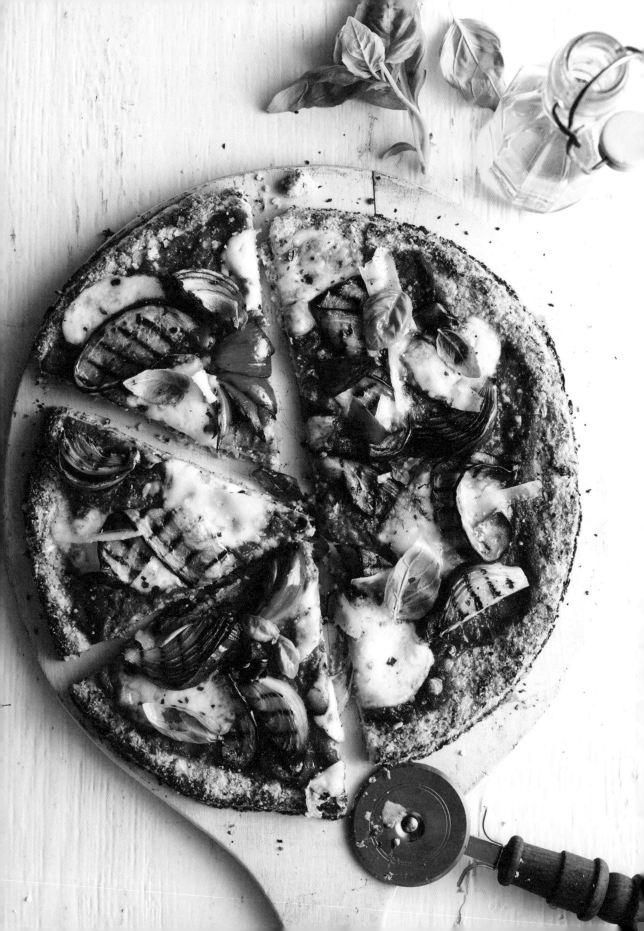

Nutrients often work more effectively together – one such partnership is vitamins C and E. Vitamin E is a fat-soluble vitamin, so it's best absorbed when eaten with some fat or oil, which helps strengthen our immune system. Vitamin C helps regenerate vitamin E so it can continue its protective role. Avocados are naturally rich in vitamin E and of course being a source of healthy fats makes them the ideal means for us to access and absorb their vitamin E content. We've combined them with vitamin C rich sweetcorn in our Peruvian chicken, avocado & quinoa salad (page 32). Another fat-soluble vitamin that supports the integrity of your immune system is vitamin A. We need vitamin A to maintain the healthy, protective linings of our nasal passage and respiratory system. Check out our recipes with orange-coloured fruits and vegetables such as Roast chicken & roots (page 30) – these veg are rich in beta-carotene, which our bodies convert to vitamin A.

Zinc is a key nutrient for strengthening our immunity and studies also suggest that, if we do catch a cold, it may help shorten the duration of it. Meat, cheese and seafood are good sources but so too are mushrooms – see our Squash, mushroom & gorgonzola pilaf on page 70.

Once you've completed the 7 days you may wish to start to build your own immunity plan using the additional recipes in this chapter – all our recipes are packed with key ingredients bursting with vitamins, minerals and phytonutrients as well as gut-friendly pre and probiotic foods, which support the health of your gut and the effectiveness of your immune function.

The secret to the success of any approach to healthy eating is preparation and planning, so we recommend using the Saturday before you start to do the shopping as well as a little bit of food prep.

We suggest you enjoy the meals as set out in the 7-day immune support chart for the most nutritionally balanced approach, but if you do want to mix, match or repeat dishes, you'll still get all the benefits of eating unprocessed and wholesome foods.

THE 7-DAY HEALTH OVERHAUL PLAN (Serves 2)

	BREAKFAST	LUNCH	SUPPER
Sunday	poached eggs with broccoli, tomatoes & wholemeal flatbread	roast chicken & roots	red pepper houmous with crispbread snaps
Monday	raspberry & almond granola	peruvian chicken, avocado & quinoa salad (using leftover chicken from sunday)	moroccan fish stew
Tuesday	bircher muesli with apple & banana	minted pea, goat's cheese & spinach wraps	sweet potato dhal with curried vegetables
Wednesday	poached eggs with broccoli, tomatoes & wholemeal flatbread	chunky vegetable & brown rice soup (freeze leftovers for later in the week)	moroccan fish stew
Thursday	raspberry & almond granola	avocado, labneh, roasted carrots & leaves	one-pot chicken with quinoa
Friday	poached eggs with broccoli, tomatoes & wholemeal flatbread	chunky vegetable & brown rice soup	steak & sweet potato chips
Saturday	bircher muesli with apple & banana	pan-fried mackerel fillets with beetroot & fennel	lamb dopiaza with broccoli rice

Poached Eggs with Broccoli, Tomatoes & Wholemeal Flatbread

Studies have shown that people who eat eggs for breakfast consume about 200 calories less at lunch than those who chose a low-protein, high carb breakfast. From an immune perspective they are a good source of vitamin A.

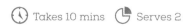 Takes 10 mins   Serves 2

- 100g/4oz thin-stemmed broccoli, trimmed and halved
- 200g/7oz cherry tomatoes on the vine
- 4 medium eggs
- 2 Wholemeal flatbreads (page 272)
- 2 tsp mixed seeds (such as sunflower, pumpkin, sesame and linseed)
- 1 tsp rapeseed oil
- good pinch of chilli flakes

1 Boil the kettle. Heat oven to 120C/100C fan/gas ½ and put an ovenproof plate inside to warm up. Fill a wide-based saucepan one-third full of water from the kettle and bring to the boil. Add the broccoli and cook for 2 mins. Add the tomatoes, return to the boil and cook for 30 secs. Lift out with tongs or a slotted spoon and place on the warm plate in the oven while you poach the eggs.

2 Return the water to a gentle simmer. Break the eggs into the pan, one at a time, and cook for 2½-3 mins or until the whites are set and the yolks are runny.

3 Divide the flatbreads between the 2 plates and top with the broccoli and tomatoes. Use a slotted spoon to drain the eggs, then place on top. Sprinkle with the seeds and drizzle with the oil. Season with a little black pepper and the chilli flakes, and serve immediately.

BENEFITS *vegetarian • folate • fibre • vit c • iron • 2 of 5 a day*
PER SERVING *383 kcals • fat 17g • saturates 4g • carbs 31g • sugars 4g • fibre 9g • protein 22g • salt 0.4g*

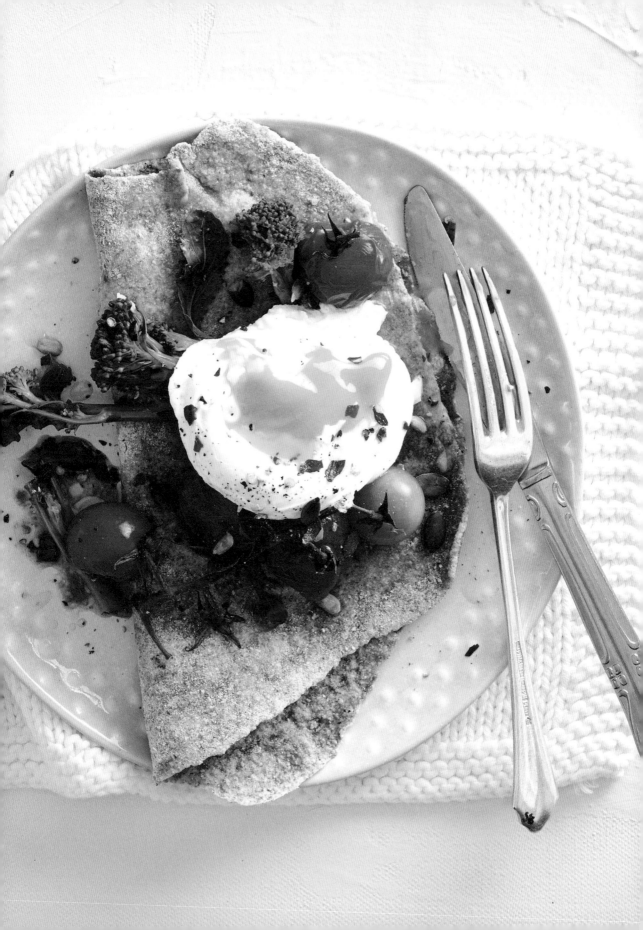

Raspberry & Almond Granola

For a dairy-free homemade oat milk to serve with this see page 9.

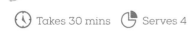

🕐 Takes 30 mins   🥧 Serves 4

- juice 2 oranges (150ml/¼ pint), plus zest of ½
- 200g/7oz jumbo rolled oats
- 1 tsp ground cinnamon
- 2 tbsp freeze-dried raspberries, or strawberries or sultanas
- 25g/1oz toasted flaked almonds
- 25g/1oz mixed seeds (such as sunflower, pumpkin, sesame and linseed)
- oat or dairy milk, to serve
- 2 oranges, peeled and cut into segments
- mint leaves (optional)

1 Heat oven to 200C/180C fan/gas 6 and line a baking tray with baking parchment. Put the orange juice in a medium saucepan and bring to the boil. Boil rapidly for 5 mins or until the liquid has reduced by half, stirring occasionally.

2 Mix the oats with the orange zest and cinnamon. Remove the pan from the heat and stir the oat mixture into the juice. Spread over the lined tray in a thin layer and bake for 10-15 mins or until lightly browned and crisp, turning the oats every few mins. Leave to cool on the tray.

3 Once cool, mix the oats with your choice of dried fruit, the flaked almonds and seeds. This can be kept in a sealed jar for up to 1 week. To serve, spoon the granola into bowls, pour over the milk and top with the orange segments and mint leaves, if you like.

BENEFITS vegetarian • folate • fibre • vit c • 1 of 5 a day
PER SERVING 305 kcals • fat 10g • saturates 1g • carbs 37g • sugars 8g • fibre 7g • protein 12g • salt 0g

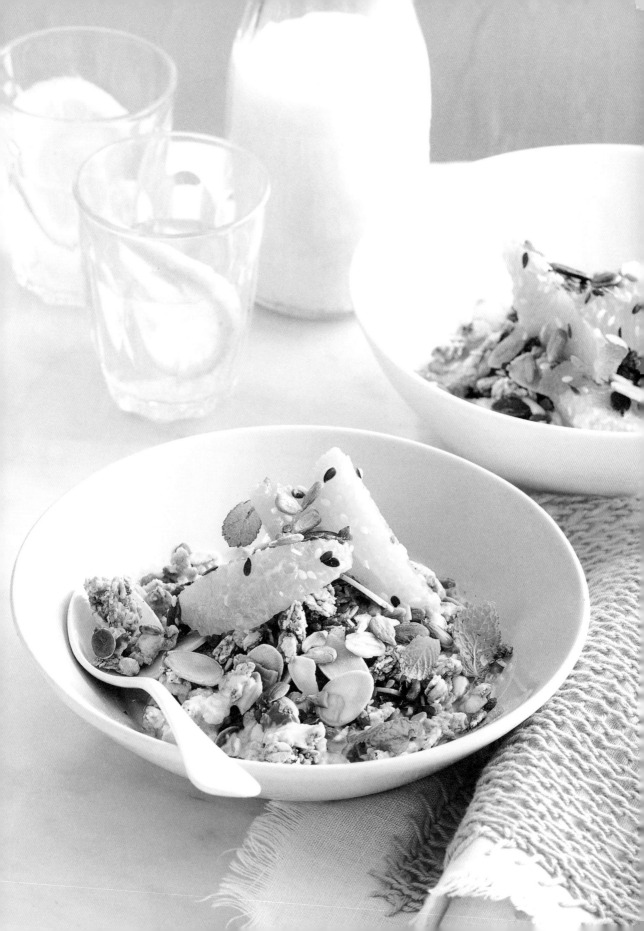

Bircher Muesli with Apple & Banana

Soaking oats and seeds overnight makes them easier to digest, and the muesli will be extra creamy - great for a quick breakfast straight from the fridge.

Takes 5 mins, plus chilling   Serves 2

- 1 eating apple, coarsely grated
- 50g/2oz jumbo rolled oats
- 25g/1oz mixed seeds (such as sunflower, pumpkin, sesame and linseed)
- 25g/1oz mixed nuts (such as Brazils, hazelnuts, almonds, pecans and walnuts), roughly chopped
- ¼ tsp ground cinnamon
- 100g/4oz bio live yogurt
- 1 medium banana, peeled and sliced
- 25g/1oz sultanas

1 Put the grated apple in a bowl and add the oats, seeds, half the nuts and the cinnamon. Toss together well. Stir in the yogurt and 100ml/3½fl oz cold water, cover and chill for several hours or overnight.
2 Spoon the muesli into 2 bowls and top with the sliced banana, sultanas and remaining nuts.

BENEFITS vegetarian • fibre • 1 of 5 a day
PER SERVING 405 kcals • fat 18g • saturates 3g • carbs 44g • sugars 28g • fibre 7g • protein 13g • salt 0.1g

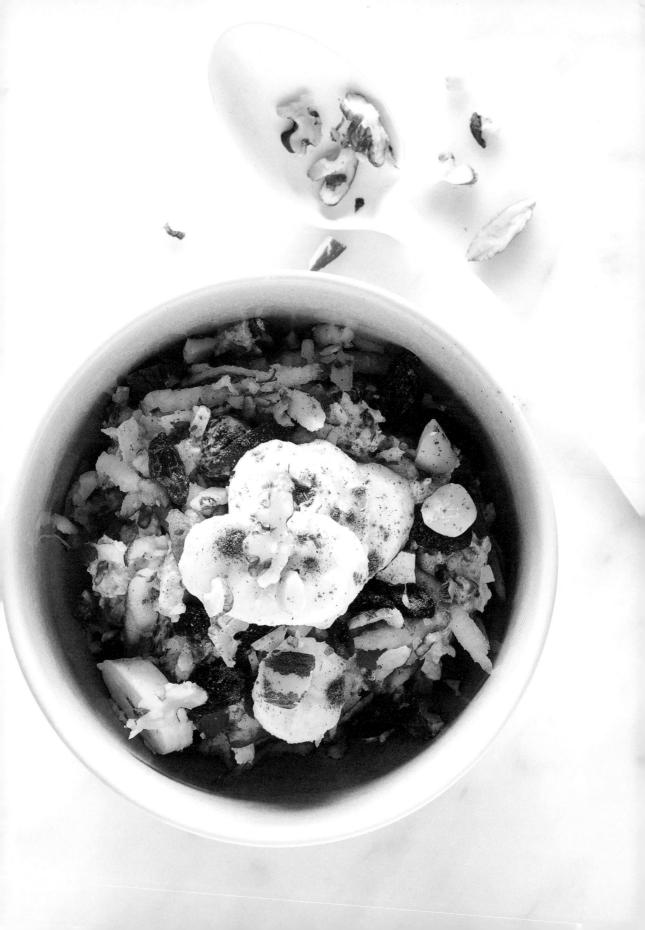

Porridge with Pear, Cinnamon & Walnuts

Oats contain a compound called beta-glucan, which not only manages cholesterol levels in the body but has an immune-supportive effect as well.

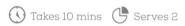 Takes 10 mins Serves 2

- 6 tbsp porridge oats
- 2 x 150g pots bio live yogurt
- 2 ripe pears, cored, skin left on and sliced
- few pinches of ground cinnamon
- small handful roughly chopped walnuts

1 Tip 400ml/14fl oz water into a small non-stick pan, stir in the oats and cook over a low heat until bubbling and thickened. You can make this in a microwave, but use 2 deep bowls to prevent spillage because the mixture will rise up as it cooks. Each bowl will take 3 mins on High.
2 Stir in the yogurt, spoon into a bowl, then top with the pear, cinnamon and walnuts.

BENEFITS vegetarian • calcium • fibre • 1 of 5 a day
PER SERVING 373 kcals • fat 14g • saturates 4g • carbs 44g • sugars 27g • fibre 11g • protein 15g • salt 0.4g

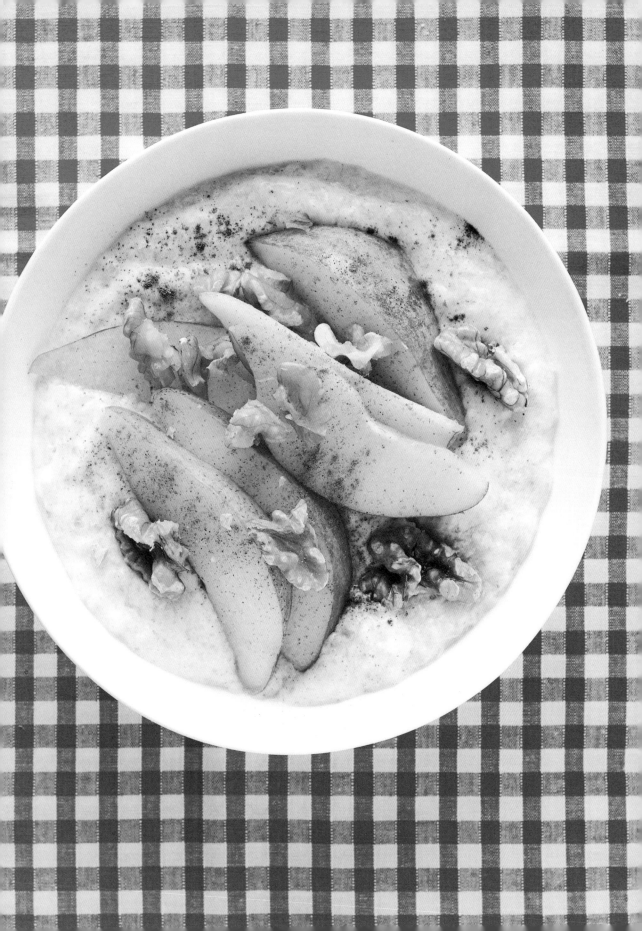

Turmeric Smoothie Bowl

A great breakfast when you are in a hurry. The oats act as slow-releasing energy, and the cashew butter is a great source of protein. Coconut contains a fat called lauric acid, which inhibits bacteria and viruses.

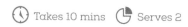 Takes 10 mins   Serves 2

- 2 tsp ground turmeric
- 3 tbsp coconut milk yogurt (we used Co Yo), or the cream skimmed from the top of canned coconut milk
- 50g/2oz porridge oats
- 1 tbsp cashew butter (or a handful of cashews)
- 2 bananas, peeled and roughly chopped
- ½ tsp ground cinnamon
- 1 tbsp chia seeds or chopped nuts, to serve

1 Put all ingredients in a blender with 600ml/1 pint water and blend until smooth. Serve in a bowl with chia seeds or some chopped nuts sprinkled over.

BENEFITS vegan • 1 of 5 a day
PER SERVING 291 kcals • fat 10g • saturates 4g • carbs 40g • sugars 20g • fibre 5g • protein 7g • salt 0g

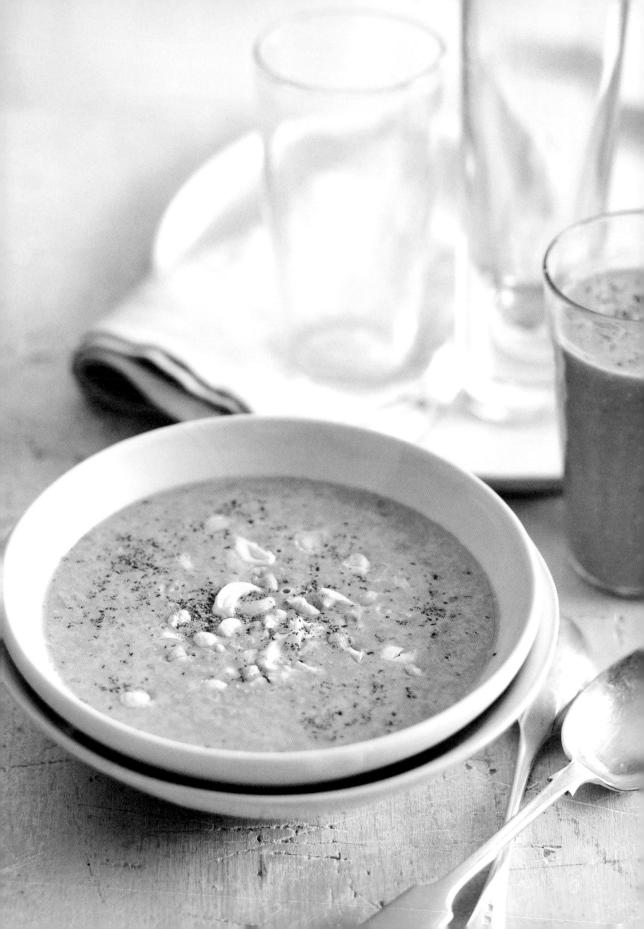

Roast Chicken & Roots

It's well worth roasting a large chicken as the leftover meat is ideal for making a salad later in the week.

 Takes 1 hour 45 mins   Serves 4

- 1.6kg/3lb 8oz whole chicken
- zest and juice 1 lemon
- 2 tbsp rapeseed oil
- 4-5 thyme sprigs, leaves roughly chopped
- 500g/1lb 2oz butternut squash, cut into chunks
- 300g/11oz carrots, cut into chunks
- 300g/11oz parsnips, peeled and cut into long batons
- 1 medium red onion, cut into thin wedges
- 1 garlic bulb, cloves separated
- 100g/4oz baby spinach leaves

1 Heat oven to 200C/180C fan/gas 6. Put the chicken in a large roasting tin. Remove any trussing elastic and retie the chicken's legs with string, if you like. Rub the lemon juice into the chicken, then rub in 1 tbsp of the oil and sprinkle with the thyme and plenty of seasoning. Roast for 25 mins.

2 Mix the squash, carrots, parsnips and onion in a bowl with the remaining oil, lemon zest and plenty of ground black pepper, and toss together well.

3 Take the chicken out of the oven and put on a plate. Scatter the vegetables into the tin, nestling the garlic cloves underneath, then put the chicken on top. Return to the oven for a further 45 mins, turning the veg after 20 mins until the chicken is cooked and the vegetables are tender and lightly browned.

4 Take the chicken out and place on a warmed platter. Cover with foil and leave to rest for 10 mins. Cook the spinach in a saucepan with a drizzle of water, and season with black pepper. Scatter the vegetables around the chicken and serve with the spinach. Squeeze the garlic out of the skins and smear over the chicken, if you like.

TIP Don't waste the chicken carcass. Use it to make and freeze an immune-boosting Bone broth, full of important minerals (page 52).

BENEFITS folate • fibre • vit c • 4 of 5 a day • gluten free
PER SERVING 524 kcals • fat 24g • saturates 5g • carbs 28g • sugars 17g • fibre 11g • protein 42g • salt 0.5g

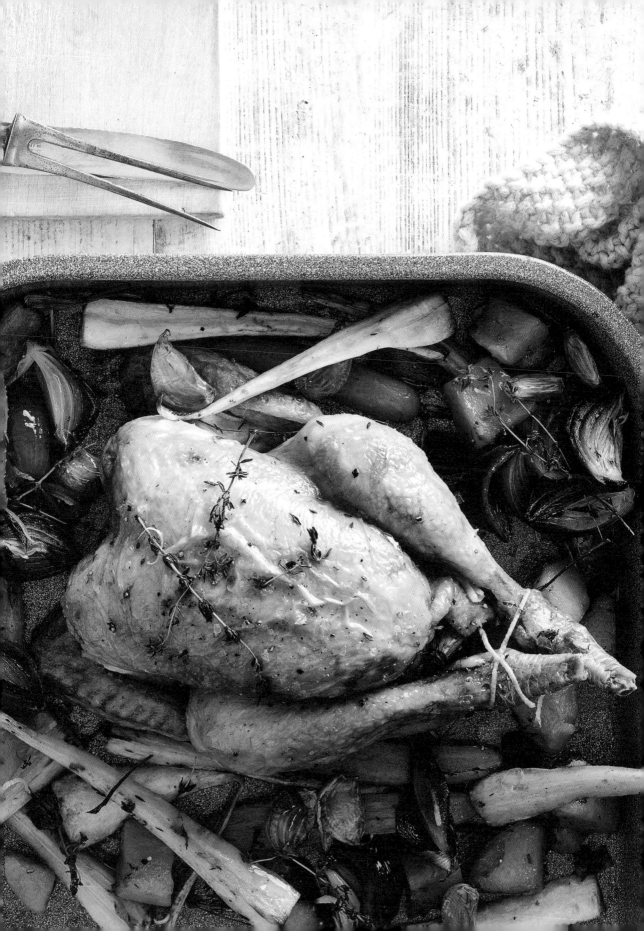

Peruvian Chicken, Avocado & Quinoa Salad

Frozen sweetcorn is a great standby ingredient – it adds colour, fibre and flavour to any dish, especially when toasted in a pan. As well as being rich in vitamin C, limes help the liver to detoxify the body, the zest is particularly potent.

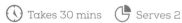 Takes 30 mins   Serves 2

- 50g/2oz uncooked quinoa
- 100g/4oz frozen sweetcorn
- 1 tbsp extra virgin rapeseed or olive oil
- 75g/2½oz cherry tomatoes, quartered
- small pack coriander, leaves roughly chopped
- 2 spring onions, trimmed and finely sliced
- zest and juice 1 lime
- ½ long red chilli, finely chopped (deseeded if you don't like it too hot)
- 1 ripe but firm avocado
- 200g/7oz skinless, cold, home cooked roast chicken, cut into chunky pieces

1 Half-fill a medium pan with water and bring to the boil. Rinse the quinoa in a fine sieve, then add to the water, stir well and simmer for 12 mins or until just tender.

2 While the quinoa is cooking, put the sweetcorn in a dry frying pan over a medium-high heat. Cook for 5 mins, turning every now and then, until defrosted and lightly toasted. Set aside.

3 Rinse the cooked quinoa in a sieve under cold water, then press hard with a serving spoon to remove excess water.

4 Tip the quinoa into a bowl and toss with the olive oil, sweetcorn, tomatoes, coriander, spring onions, lime zest and chilli. Season well with black pepper.

5 Halve and stone the avocado. Scoop out the flesh with a large metal spoon, cut into slices and combine with the lime juice. Add the chicken pieces and avocado to the salad and toss gently together before serving.

BENEFITS *vit c • 2 of 5 a day • gluten free*
PER SERVING *512 kcals • fat 29g • saturates 6g • carbs 26g • sugars 5g • fibre 5g • protein 34g • salt 0.3g*

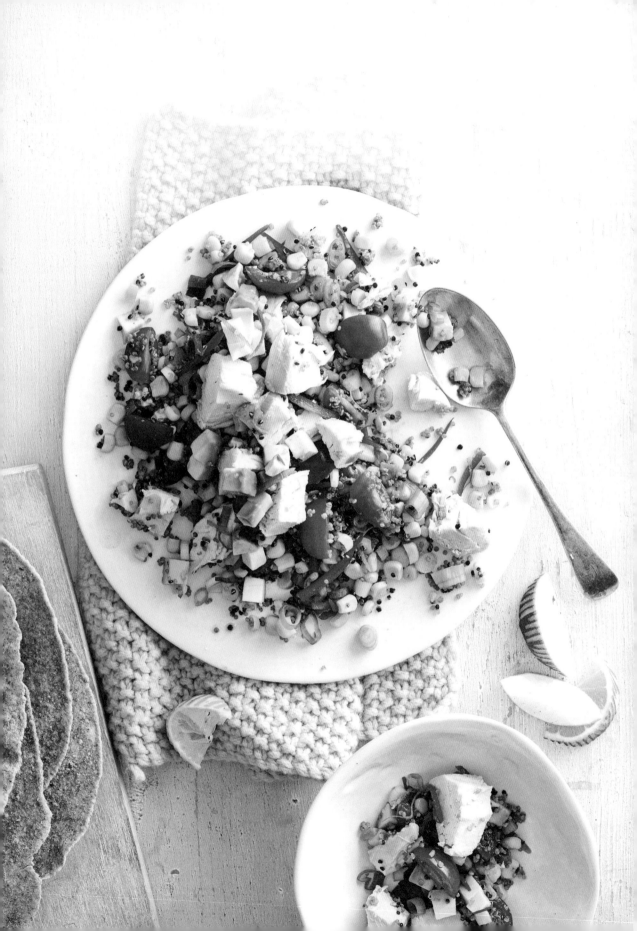

Minted Pea, Goat's Cheese & Spinach Wraps

These wraps are loaded with immune-friendly nutrients, including vitamin C. Out of season, frozen vegetables are great to use instead of fresh because they're picked at their peak and frozen immediately to lock in the goodness.

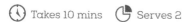 Takes 10 mins Serves 2

- 140g/5oz frozen peas, thawed
- ½ small pack mint, finely chopped
- finely grated zest 1 lemon
- 75g/2½oz soft rindless goat's cheese log
- 2 Wholemeal flatbreads (page 272)
- 50g/2oz baby spinach leaves
- 1 apple, coarsely grated
- 25g/1oz mixed seeds, such as linseed, sunflower, pumpkin and sesame

1 Put the peas in a bowl and lightly mash with the mint, lemon zest and goat's cheese. Season well with ground black pepper. Keep chilled if not serving straight away.
2 Spread each flatbread with the pea and goat's cheese mixture, then top with the spinach, apple and seeds. Roll up and serve immediately, or wrap in foil and pop into a packed lunch. Can be made the night before.

BENEFITS vegetarian • folate • vit c • iron • 2 of 5 a day • fibre
PER SERVING 457 kcals • fat 19g • saturates 8g • carbs 42g • sugars 10g • fibre 14g • protein 22g • salt 0.7g

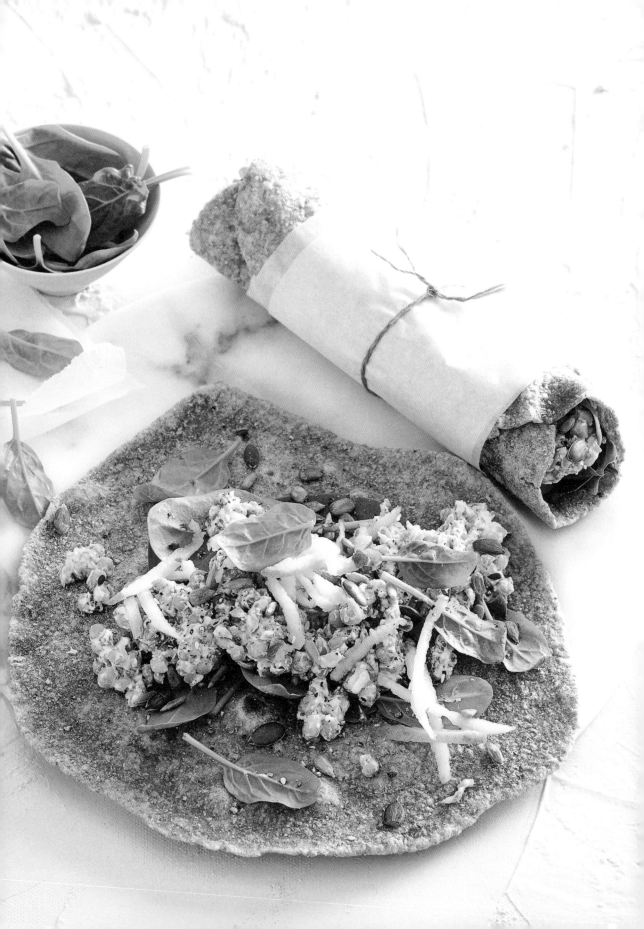

Chunky Vegetable & Brown Rice Soup

This makes four portions, so you could serve this soup chunky one day and puréed the next if you like.

🕐 Takes 1 hour 10 mins   ◔ Serves 4

- 2 tbsp rapeseed oil
- 1 medium onion, halved and sliced
- 2 garlic cloves, finely sliced
- 2 celery sticks, trimmed and thinly sliced
- 2 medium carrots, cut into chunks
- 2 medium parsnips, cut into chunks
- 1 tbsp finely chopped thyme leaves
- 100g/4oz brown basmati rice
- 2 medium leeks, sliced
- ½ small pack parsley, to garnish

1 Heat the oil in a large non-stick pan and add the onion, garlic, celery, carrots, parsnips and thyme. Cover with a lid and cook gently for 15 mins, stirring occasionally, until the onion is softened and beginning to colour. Add the rice and pour in 1.2 litres/2 pints cold water. Bring to the boil, then reduce the heat to a simmer and cook, uncovered, for 15 mins, stirring occasionally.

2 Season the soup with plenty of ground black pepper and salt to taste, then stir in the leeks. Return to a gentle simmer and cook for a further 5 mins or until the leeks have softened. Adjust the seasoning to taste and blitz half the soup with a stick blender, leaving the other half chunky, if you like. Top with the parsley and serve in deep bowls.

TIP Once cool, leftovers can be stored in the fridge for up to 2 days, or covered and frozen for up to 1 month. Thaw overnight in the fridge and reheat in a saucepan until piping hot throughout.

BENEFITS vegan • folate • vit c • iron • fibre • low fat • 2 of 5 a day • gluten free
PER SERVING 261 kcals • fat 8g • saturates 1g • carbs 37g • sugars 11g • fibre 10g • protein 5g • salt 0.5g

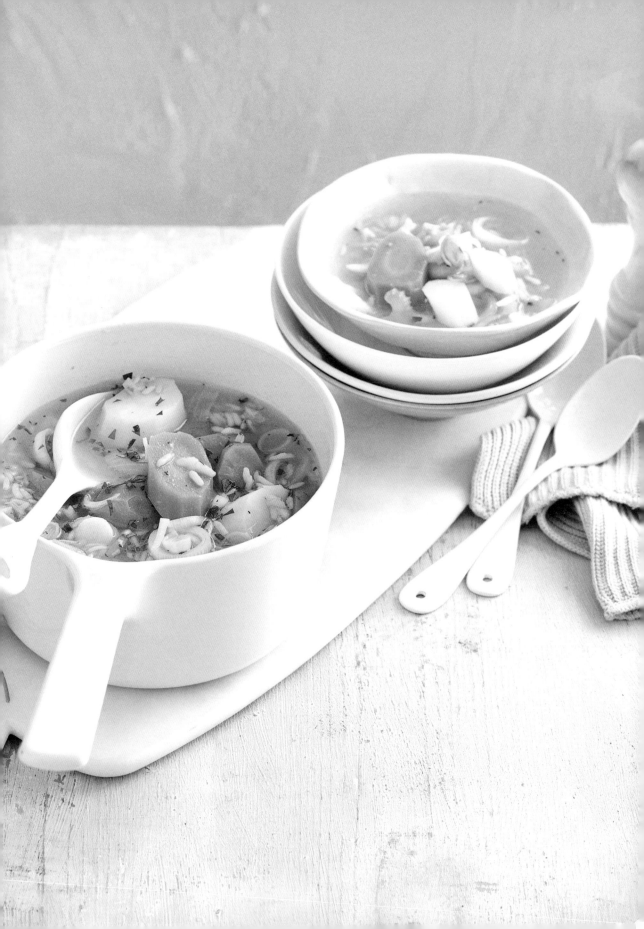

Avocado, Labneh, Roasted Carrots & Leaves

Making your own soft cheese – labneh – from bio yogurt is surprisingly easy. It's delicious in salads and wraps, as a dip with crunchy vegetables or melted into baked sweet potatoes.

Takes 50 mins, plus overnight chilling   Serves 2

- 200g/7oz bio live yogurt
- grated zest 1 lime, plus 1 tbsp juice, lime cut into wedges, to serve
- ½ small pack coriander, leaves finely chopped
- 300g/11oz carrots, cut into batons
- 1 tbsp rapeseed oil
- ½ tsp ground cumin
- 1 ripe but firm avocado
- 50g bag mixed salad leaves
- 1 tbsp mixed seeds (such as sunflower, pumpkin, sesame and linseed)

1 To make the labneh, mix the yogurt, lime zest and coriander together in a bowl. Line another small bowl with a square of muslin. Spoon the yogurt mixture into the bowl, pull up the ends of the muslin and tie the yogurt into a ball. Tie the ends of the muslin onto a wooden spoon and suspend over a bowl or jug. Put in the fridge overnight to strain.

2 Heat oven to 200C/180C fan/gas 6. Toss the carrots with 1 tsp of the oil, 2 tsp of the lime juice, the cumin and lots of ground black pepper. Tip onto a foil-lined baking tray and roast for 20 mins. Turn the carrots and return to the oven for a further 10 mins or until tender and lightly browned. Set aside.

3 Cut the avocado in half and remove the stone. Scoop out the flesh from each half in one piece with a serving spoon. Slice on a chopping board, then toss with the remaining lime juice.

4 Untie the labneh and spread it over two plates, top with the salad leaves, carrots and avocado. Drizzle over the remaining oil, sprinkle with the seeds and serve with the lime wedges.

BENEFITS *vegetarian • low cal • calcium • fibre • 3 of 5 a day • gluten free*
PER SERVING *370 kcals • fat 25g • saturates 5g • carbs 21g • sugars 19g • fibre 9g • protein 9g • salt 0.3g*

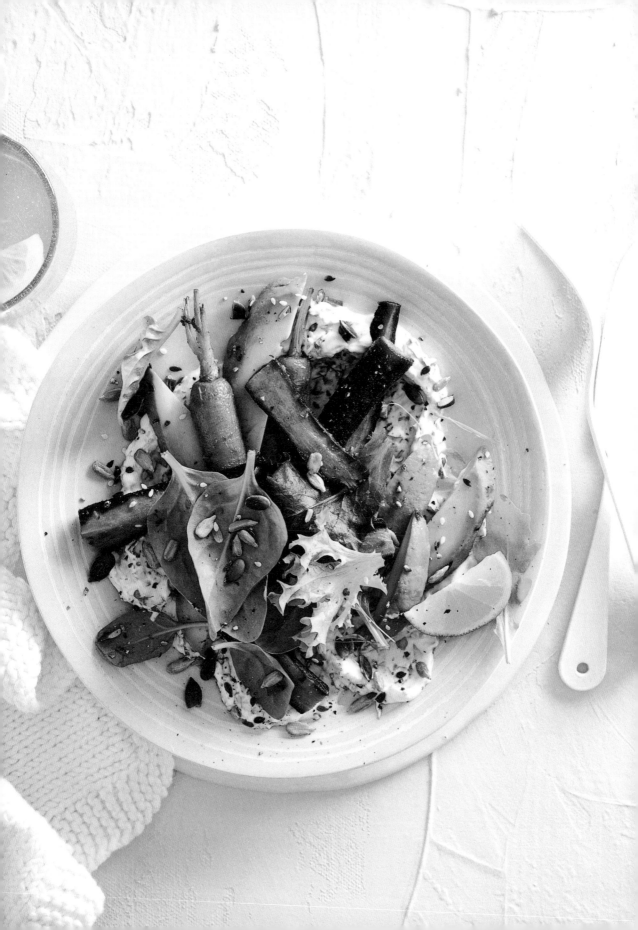

Pan-fried Mackerel Fillets with Beetroot & Fennel

Mackerel fillets contain the beneficial fats, known as omega-3. These fats help the immune system function more effectively. Mackerel is quick to cook, and really complements this earthy salad.

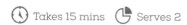 Takes 15 mins   Serves 2

- 2 mackerel fillets (about 300g/11oz)
- 2 tsp cold-pressed rapeseed or olive oil
- ½ small fennel bulb, quartered and very thinly sliced
- 1 small beetroot, peeled and very thinly sliced
- 100g/4oz cucumber, halved and thinly sliced
- 1 eating apple, cored, quartered and sliced
- 1 tbsp lemon juice, plus lemon wedges, to serve
- 100g/4oz bio live yogurt
- ½ small pack dill

1 Put one of the mackerel fillets on a board and cut a 'V' down the centre, either side of the pin bones, to create two smaller fillets, then remove the bones. Repeat with the other fillet. Rub with the oil and season with plenty of ground black pepper. Set aside.

2 Put the fennel in a bowl with the beetroot, cucumber and apple. Drizzle over the lemon juice, add the yogurt and mix well. Roughly chop the dill, putting aside a few fronds to garnish, and scatter over the salad, then season with ground black pepper and toss together lightly. Set aside.

3 Put a large non-stick frying pan over a medium-high heat. When hot, add the fish, skin-side down, and cook for 2½ mins. Flip the fish over and cook for 30 secs on the other side.

4 Put the fillets on top of the salad and serve with the dill fronds and lemon wedges for squeezing over.

BENEFITS low cal • folate • vit c • 2 of 5 a day • gluten free • omega 3
PER SERVING 397 kcals • fat 24g • saturates 5g • carbs 15g • sugars 15g • fibre 5g • protein 27g • salt 0.4g

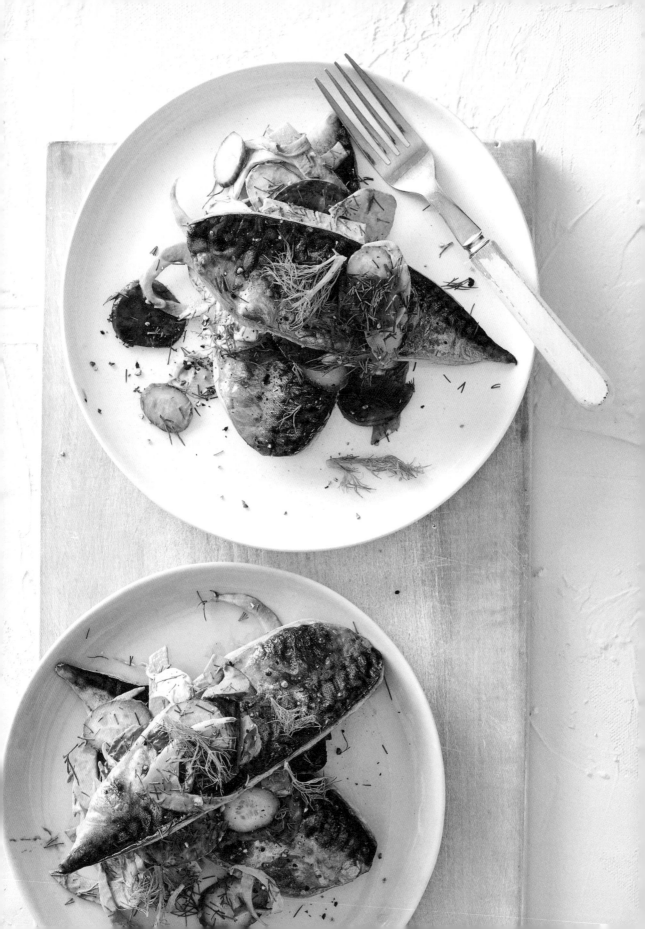

Roast Squash & Kale Salad with Orange Dressing

This tastes fresh and full of interesting flavours and textures. The active oils in garlic work like an antibiotic, so are helpful for treating infections.

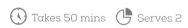 Takes 50 mins   Serves 2

- 2 red onions, each cut into 4 thick slices
- 4 garlic cloves, unpeeled
- 8 small wedges of butternut squash (prepared weight 250g/9oz)
- 2 tsp rapeseed oil
- ½ tsp caraway or fennel seeds
- ½ x 60g bag baby kale or rocket
- 50g/2oz pomegranate seeds (about ¼ of a large fruit)
- 50g/2oz feta, crumbled

FOR THE DRESSING
- 1 orange
- 1 tbsp apple cider vinegar
- 1 tsp rapeseed oil
- 2 tbsp pumpkin seeds

1 Heat oven to 200C/180C fan/gas 6. Toss the onions, garlic and squash in the oil, then arrange in a single layer on a baking tray and roast for 25 mins.

2 Remove the garlic and set aside, turn the veg over with a fish slice, sprinkle over the caraway or fennel and return to the oven for 10 mins more.

3 To make the dressing, pare the zest from half the orange and put in a bowl. Cut the peel and pith from the orange with a sharp knife. Working over the bowl to catch the juices, cut out the segments from between the membrane. Stir in the vinegar, oil and pumpkin seeds. Discard the skin of the roasted garlic, mash the soft cloves and add to the bowl. Stir well.

4 Pile the roasted veg onto a platter or plates, top with the kale, then spoon over the dressing and toss. Scatter over the pomegranate seeds and feta, and serve.

BENEFITS vegetarian • low cal • calcium • folate • fibre • vit c • 3 of 5 a day • gluten free
PER SERVING 360 kcals • fat 17g • saturates 5g • carbs 24g • sugars 22g • fibre 8g • protein 13g • salt 1g

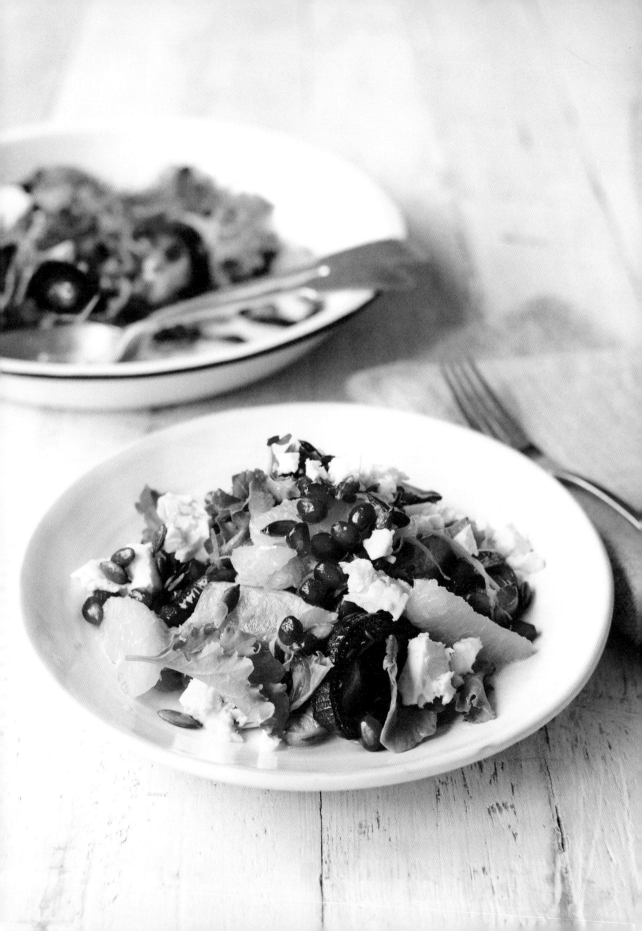

Veggie Tahini Lentils

Quick, easy and packed with healthy gut-friendly veg, this is a great midweek meal.

🕐 Takes 20 mins   ◔ Serves 4

- 100g/4oz Puy lentils
- 50g/2oz tahini
- zest and juice 1 lemon
- 2 tbsp rapeseed oil
- 1 red onion, thinly sliced
- 1 garlic clove, crushed
- 1 yellow pepper, thinly sliced
- 200g/8oz green beans, trimmed and halved
- 1 courgette, sliced into half moons
- 100g/4oz shredded kale

1 Boil the lentils according to pack instructions then drain. Meanwhile mix the tahini with the zest and juice of the lemon and 50ml/2fl oz of cold water to make a runny dressing. Season to taste, then set aside.

2 Heat the oil in a wok or large frying pan over a medium-high heat. Add the red onion, and fry for 2 mins until starting to soften and colour. Add the garlic, yellow pepper, green beans and the courgette and fry for 5 mins, stirring frequently.

3 Tip in the kale, lentils and the tahini dressing. Keep the pan on the heat for a couple of mins, stirring everything together until the kale is wilted and it's all coated in the creamy dressing. This will keep in the fridge for a couple of days, reheat in a pan with a dash of water.

BENEFITS vegan • low cal • folate • fibre • vit c • 3 of 5 a day • gluten free
PER SERVING 293 kcals • fat 14g • saturates 2g • carbs 23g • sugars 7g • fibre 10g • protein 13g • salt 0.7g

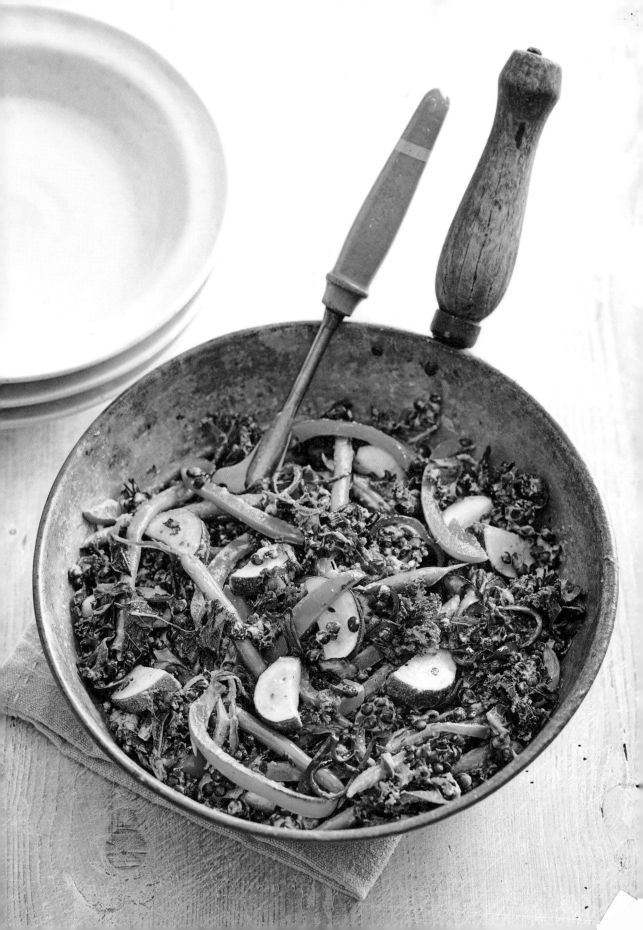

Egg & Puy Lentil Salad
with Tamari & Watercress

The carrot in this, and other orange-coloured veg like sweet potato, is rich in carotenoids, which our bodies convert to vitamin A - vital for a healthy respiratory system.

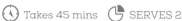 Takes 45 mins   SERVES 2

- 175g/6oz cauliflower florets, broken into smaller pieces
- 1 tbsp rapeseed oil, plus a drizzle
- 75g/2½oz Puy lentils
- 1 large carrot, chopped into small pieces
- 2 celery sticks, chopped into small pieces
- 2 garlic cloves
- 3 eggs
- 1 tbsp wheat-free tamari
- 10 cherry tomatoes, halved
- 4 spring onions, finely sliced
- 2 generous handfuls watercress, large stems removed

1 Heat oven to 220C/200C fan/gas 7. Toss the cauliflower with a drizzle of the oil, then roast for 20 mins on a parchment-lined baking tray until tender and tinged with gold round the edges.

3 Meanwhile, put the lentils in a pan with the carrot and celery. Pour in water to cover, put on a lid and boil for 20 mins until the lentils are tender. Check before they are ready in case they are boiling dry and, if necessary, top up with a little more water.

4 While they are cooking, finely grate the garlic and set aside in a large bowl, and boil the eggs for 6 mins. This will give you eggs with a soft yolk. When they are ready, plunge into cold water, then shell.

5 Mix the tamari and oil into the garlic to make a dressing. Check the lentils and drain, if necessary, then toss in the bowl with the dressing, tomatoes, spring onions, cauliflower and watercress. Pile onto a plate and top with the eggs, adding any remaining dressing from the bowl over the top.

BENEFITS *vegetarian • low cal • calcium • folate • fibre • vit c • iron • 4 of 5 a day • gluten free*
PER SERVING *411 kcals • fat 18g • saturates 3g • carbs 30g • sugars 11g • fibre 12g • protein 26g • salt 1.6g*

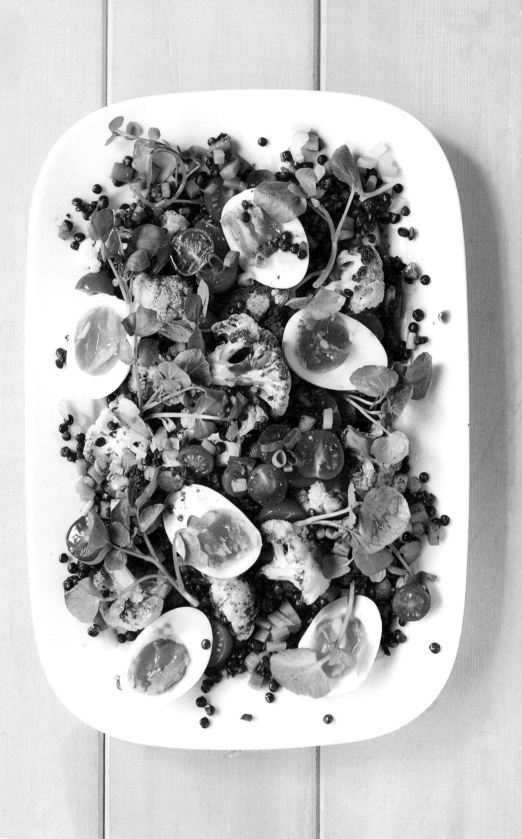

Mushroom & Basil Omelette with Grilled Tomatoes

This makes an easy vegetarian lunch or brunch for two to share. Serve the omelette and tomatoes on their own or with a crisp green salad.

🕐 Takes 20 minutes   ◔ Serves 2

- 2 tomatoes, halved
- 3 medium eggs
- 1 tbsp snipped chives
- 1 tsp unsalted butter
- 300g/11oz chestnut mushrooms, sliced
- 2 tbsp soft cheese
- 1 tbsp finely torn basil leaves
- green salad, to serve (optional)

1 Heat grill to high and grill the tomatoes, turning occasionally to prevent burning, until slightly scorched. Keep warm.

2 Beat the eggs in a bowl, add a small splash of water and mix. Add the chives and some black pepper, and beat again. Set aside.

3 In a non-stick frying pan, heat the butter over a medium heat until foaming. Cook the mushrooms for 5–8 mins until tender, stirring occasionally. Remove and set aside.

4 Briskly stir the egg mixture, then add to the hot pan (tilting it so that the mixture covers the entire base). Leave for 10 seconds or so until it begins to set, then gently stir to cook any unset egg.

5 Spoon the mushroom mix to one side of the omelette, and top with the cheese and basil. Flip the omelette, if you like. Cook for 1 min more, cut in half and slide on to plates. Serve with the tomatoes and a green salad, if you like.

BENEFITS *vegetarian • low cal • folate • 2 of 5 a day*
PER SERVING *205 kcals • fat 14g • saturates 6g • carbs 4g • sugars 4g • fibre 3g • protein 15g • salt 0.5g*

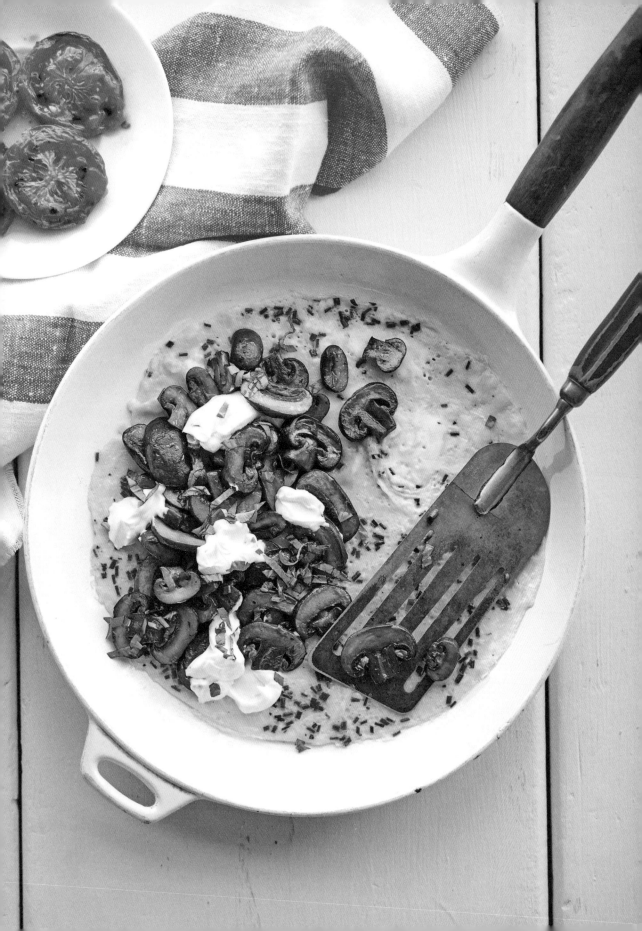

Beef Goulash Soup

This meal in a bowl is packed with 3 of your 5 a day. Don't omit the topping as the parsley contributes to the vitamin C, while the bio yogurt is good for the gut.

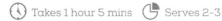 Takes 1 hour 5 mins   Serves 2-3

- 1 tbsp rapeseed oil
- 1 large onion, halved and sliced
- 3 garlic cloves, sliced
- 200g/7oz lean stewing beef, finely diced
- 1 tsp caraway seeds
- 2 tsp smoked paprika
- 400g can chopped tomatoes
- 600ml/1 pint vegetable bouillon or beef stock
- 1 medium sweet potato, peeled and diced
- 1 green pepper, deseeded and diced

FOR TOPPING
- 150g pot bio live yogurt
- good handful chopped parsley

1 Heat the oil in a large pan, add the onion and garlic and fry for 5 mins until starting to colour. Stir in the beef, increase the heat and fry, stirring, to brown it.
2 Add the caraway and paprika, stir well, then tip in the tomatoes and stock. Cover and leave to cook gently for 30 mins.
3 Stir in the sweet potato and green pepper, cover the pan again and cook for 20 mins more or until tender. Allow to cool a little, then serve topped with the yogurt and chopped parsley.

BENEFITS low fat • low cal • fibre • vit c • 3 of 5 a day
PER SERVING (3) 345 kcals • fat 12g • saturates 4g • carbs 28g • sugars 18g • fibre 7g • protein 25g • salt 1g

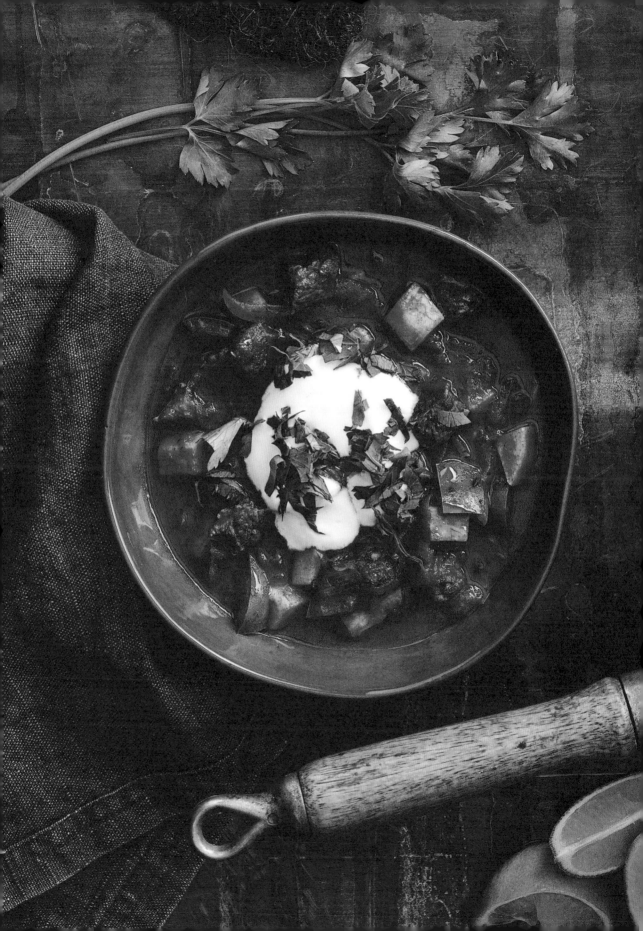

Bone Broth

Don't throw away a chicken carcass, it makes a really nourishing soup full of amino acids, gelatin (good for the joints) and minerals like selenium and zinc, which are key to a healthy immune function.

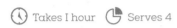 Takes 1 hour   Serves 4

- 1 meaty leftover chicken carcass, skin removed
- 1 large onion, halved and sliced
- grated zest and juice 1 lemon
- 2 bay leaves, fresh or dried
- 1-2 red chillies, halved, deseeded and sliced
- 1 tsp ground coriander
- ½ tsp ground cumin
- small pack fresh coriander, stems and leaves chopped but kept apart
- 1 large garlic clove, finely grated
- 250g/9oz cooked brown basmati rice

1 Break the chicken carcass into a large pan, then add the onion, 1.5 litres/2½ pints water, the lemon juice and bay leaves. Cover the pan and simmer for 40 mins. Remove from the heat and allow it to cool slightly.

2 Place a colander over a bowl, then scoop out all of the bones into the colander and pick through them, stripping off the chicken and returning it to the pan with any onion as you work your way down the pile of bones.

3 Return any broth from the bowl to the pan with the chillies, ground coriander, cumin, fresh coriander stems, lemon zest and garlic and cook for a few mins until just bubbling. Don't boil hard as you will spoil the delicate flavours. Season only if you need to.

4 Meanwhile, heat the rice according to the pack and toss with the chopped coriander leaves. Ladle the broth into bowls, top with the rice and serve.

BENEFITS *low fat • gluten free*
PER SERVING *150 kcals • fat 3g • saturates 1g • carbs 24g • sugars 5g • fibre 2g • protein 6g, salt 0.9g*

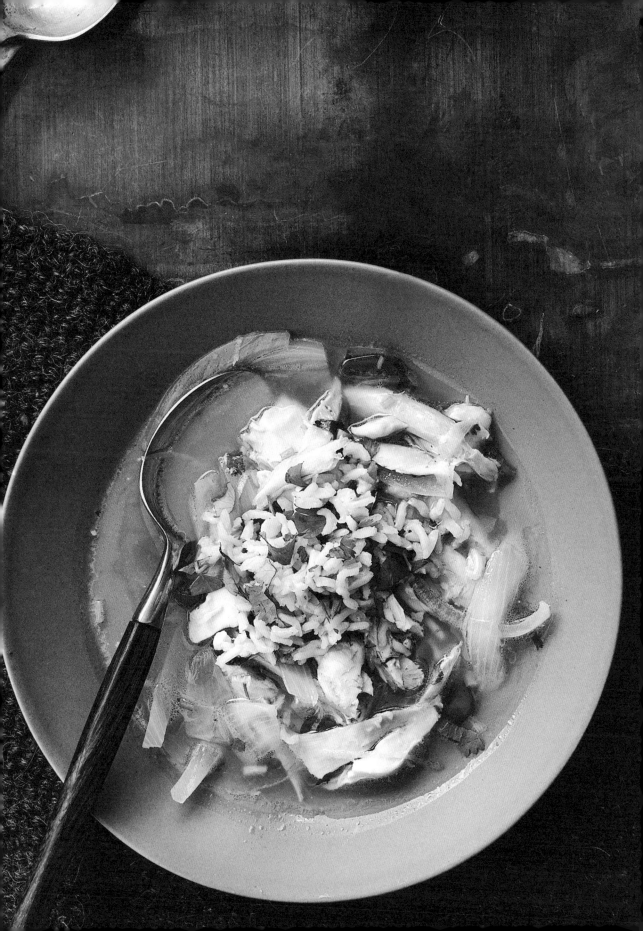

Chicken, Broccoli & Beetroot Salad with Avocado Pesto

This really is the ultimate lunch – it's packed with protein and other ingredients that give your body a boost like the healthy fats from the avocado and antioxidants from the broccoli.

🕐 Takes 30 mins   🕐 Serves 2

- 125g/4½oz thin-stemmed broccoli
- 1 tsp rapeseed oil
- 1½ skinless chicken breasts
- 1 small red onion, thinly sliced
- ½ a 100g bag watercress
- 1 raw beetroot, peeled and julienned or grated
- ½ tsp nigella seeds

FOR THE AVOCADO PESTO
- ½ a small pack basil
- 1 small avocado
- ½ garlic clove, crushed
- 15g/½oz walnut halves, crumbled
- ½ tbsp rapeseed oil
- juice and zest ½ lemon

1 Bring a large pan of water to the boil, add the broccoli and cook for 2 mins. Drain, then refresh under cold water. Heat a griddle pan, toss the broccoli in ½ tsp of the rapeseed oil and griddle for 2-3 mins, turning, until a little charred. Set aside to cool. Brush the chicken with the remaining oil and season. Griddle for 3-4 mins each side or until cooked through. Leave to cool, then slice or shred into chunky pieces.

2 Next, make the pesto. Pick the leaves from the basil and set aside a handful to top the salad. Put the rest in the small bowl of a food processor. Scoop the flesh from the avocado and add to the food processor with the garlic, walnuts, oil, 1 tbsp lemon juice, 2-3 tbsp cold water and some seasoning. Blitz until smooth, then transfer to a small serving dish. Pour the remaining lemon juice over the sliced onion and leave for a few mins.

3 Pile the watercress onto a large platter. Toss through the broccoli and onion, along with the lemon juice it was soaked in. Top with the beetroot, but don't mix it in, and the chicken. Scatter over the reserved basil leaves, the lemon zest and nigella seeds, then serve with the avocado pesto.

BENEFITS low cal • folate • fibre • vit c • 2 of 5 a day • gluten free
PER SERVING 320 kcals • fat 18g • saturates 3g • carbs 8g • sugars 6g • fibre 6g • protein 29g • salt 0.3g

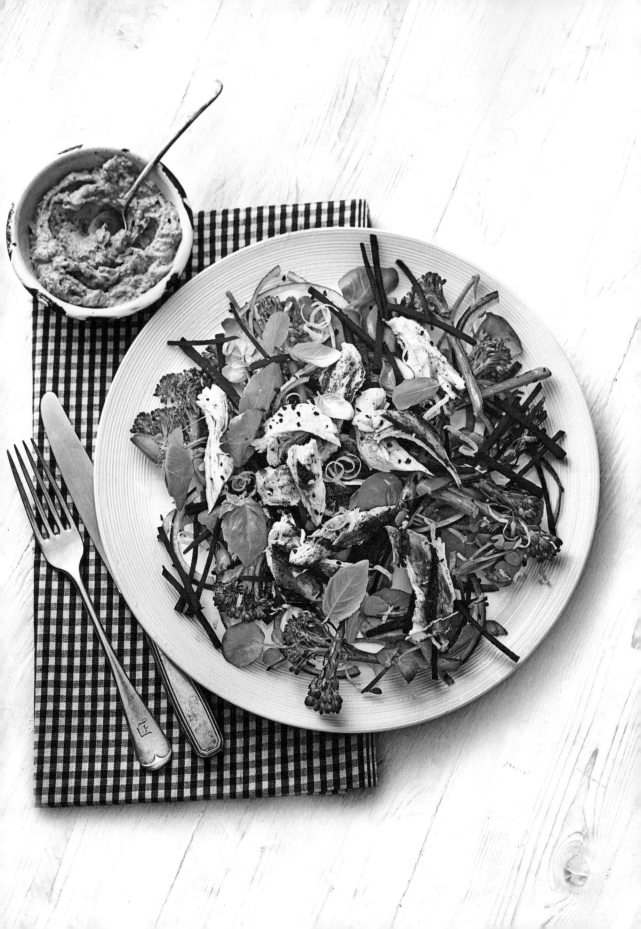

Red Pepper Houmous with Crispbread Snaps

These crunchy crispbreads are simple to prepare and will keep for a week in an airtight container. Any leftover raw veg from this diet plan will pair well with the houmous.

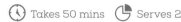 Takes 50 mins Serves 2

- 1 tsp rapeseed oil
- 1 red pepper, deseeded and sliced into thin strips
- 1 garlic clove, crushed
- ¼ tsp chilli flakes
- 400g can haricot beans, drained and rinsed
- 1 tbsp extra virgin olive oil
- 2 tbsp lemon juice
- assorted vegetable sticks, for dipping (optional – we used celery and purple carrots)

FOR THE CRISPBREAD SNAPS
- 50g/2oz wholemeal flour, plus extra for dusting
- ¼ tsp baking powder
- 1 tbsp mixed seeds (such as sunflower, pumpkin, sesame and linseed)
- 1 tbsp finely chopped thyme leaves
- 50g/2oz bio live yogurt
- ½ tsp extra virgin olive oil

1 To make the crispbread, heat oven to 190C/170C fan/ gas 5. In a bowl, mix the flour with the baking powder, seeds and thyme. Add the yogurt and mix with your hands to make a soft dough.

2 Place a sheet of baking parchment on the work surface and sprinkle with a little flour. Flour a rolling pin and roll out the dough until around 3mm/⅛in thick. You will need to turn and lift the dough, sprinkling with a little more flour as you roll so it doesn't stick.

3 Transfer the baking parchment with the dough on to a baking tray, then prick all over with a fork. Brush lightly with the oil and bake for 20-25 mins until lightly browned and dry. The dough will continue to crisp as it cools. Once cold, break into chunky pieces and store in an airtight container for up to 1 week.

4 Meanwhile, heat the rapeseed oil in a small saucepan over a medium-high heat. Add the pepper, cover with a lid and fry for 10 mins or until softened and lightly browned in places. Remove the lid every few mins and stir, adding a splash of water if the pepper begins to stick. Add the garlic and chilli flakes, and cook for a few secs more, stirring. Leave to cool for 5 mins.

5 Tip the pepper, garlic and chilli into a food processor and add the haricot beans, olive oil, lemon juice and lots of ground black pepper. Blitz until smooth, then scoop into a bowl or two lidded containers and leave to cool. Serve with the crispbread snaps and vegetable sticks, for dipping, if you like.

BENEFITS vegetarian • fibre • vit c • 2 of 5 a day
PER SERVING 346 kcals • fat 12g • saturates 2g • carbs 36g • sugars 8g • fibre 16g • protein 14g • salt 0.3g

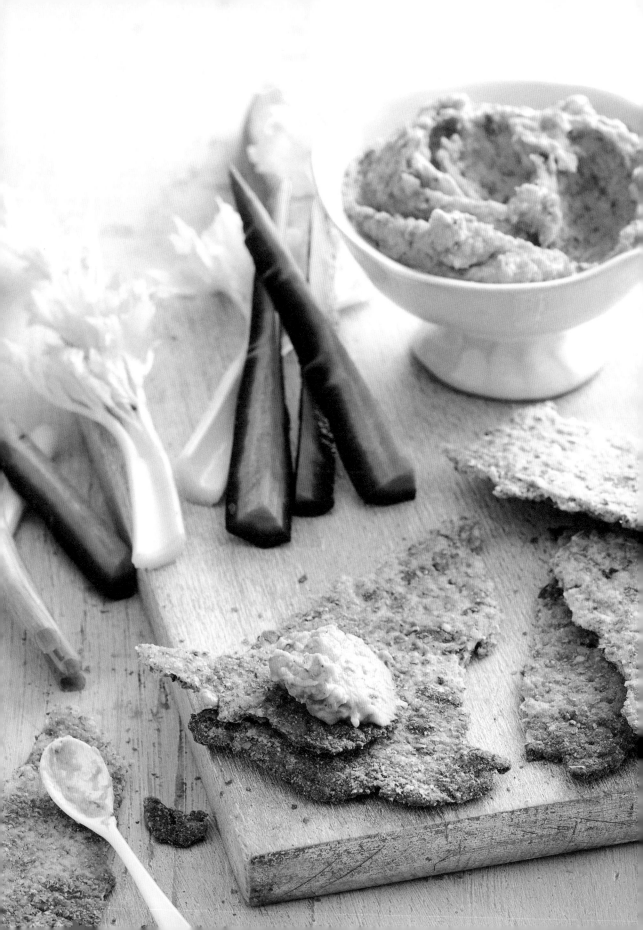

Moroccan Fish Stew

This quick and easy one-pot is bursting with gut-friendly vegetables like leeks, onion and garlic. Combining salmon, an oily fish, with sweet potatoes not only results in a healthy, filling dinner, but aids absorption of fat-soluble vitamin A.

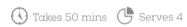 Takes 50 mins   Serves 4

- 1 tbsp rapeseed oil
- 1 onion, thinly sliced
- 2 thin leeks, trimmed and sliced
- ½ small fennel bulb, quartered and very thinly sliced
- 2 large garlic cloves, finely sliced
- 2 tsp ground coriander
- 1 tsp ground cumin
- ½ tsp chilli flakes
- ¼ tsp ground cinnamon
- 400g can chopped tomatoes
- 375g/13oz sweet potatoes, peeled and cut into chunks
- 1 yellow and 1 red pepper, deseeded and cut into chunks
- 400g can chickpeas, drained and rinsed
- juice 1 large orange, the peel thickly sliced with a vegetable peeler
- 200g/7oz skinless line-caught cod, haddock or pollock fillet, cut into chunks
- 200g/7oz skinless wild salmon, cut into chunks
- ½ small pack flat-leaf parsley, roughly chopped

1 Heat the oil in a large flameproof casserole dish or saucepan and gently fry the onion, leeks and fennel for 10 mins, stirring occasionally, or until the veg is well softened and lightly browned. Add the garlic and spices, and cook for 30 secs more. Season well with ground black pepper.

2 Tip in the chopped tomatoes, sweet potatoes, peppers, chickpeas, orange juice and peel with 300ml/½ pint water and bring to a gentle simmer. Cover loosely and cook for 20 mins, stirring occasionally, until the potatoes are softened but not breaking apart.

3 Add the fish pieces on top of the bubbling liquid and cover. Poach over a medium heat for 3-4 mins or until the fish is just cooked. Adjust the seasoning and serve scattered with parsley.

TIP If cooking for 2 people, chill the remaining 2 portions of stew after step 2, before adding the fish. It will keep for up to 2 days. When ready to serve, simply reheat the stew on the hob, and complete from step 3.

BENEFITS low fat • low cal • folate • fibre • vit c • iron • 5 of 5 a day • gluten free • omega 3
PER SERVING 448 kcals • fat 12g • saturates 2g • carbs 49g • sugars 26g • fibre 13g • protein 29g • salt 0.7g

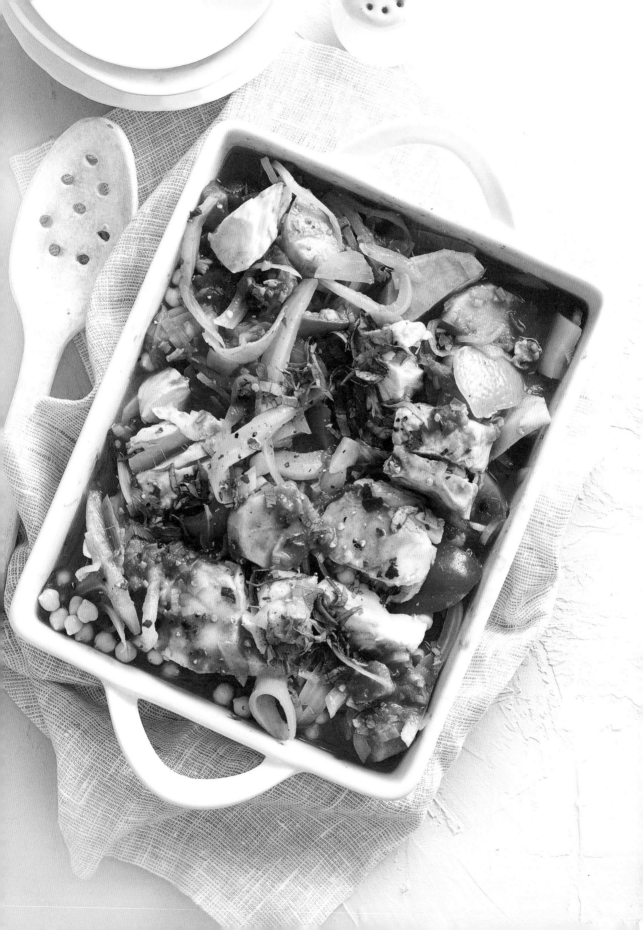

Sweet Potato Dhal with Curried Vegetables

This rich and comforting spicy dhal, topped with lightly curried vegetables, is delicious served with creamy yogurt and zesty lime.

 Takes 1 hour 35 mins   Serves 4

- 1 tbsp rapeseed oil
- 1 medium onion, finely chopped
- 2 garlic cloves, thinly sliced
- 1 tbsp medium curry powder
- 200g/7oz dried split red lentils
- 500g/1lb 2oz sweet potatoes, peeled and cut into chunks
- 2 tbsp lime (or lemon) juice, plus lime wedges, to serve
- 100g/4oz bio live yogurt
- coriander, to serve

FOR THE CURRIED VEGETABLES
- 100g/4oz green beans, trimmed and cut into short lengths
- 250g/9oz cauliflower, cut into small florets
- 2 medium carrots, sliced
- 1 tbsp rapeseed oil
- 1 onion, cut into thin wedges
- 2 garlic cloves, thinly sliced
- 1 tsp medium curry powder
- 200g/7oz ripe tomatoes, roughly chopped
- 1 long green chilli, finely sliced (deseeded if you don't like it too hot)

1 To make the dhal, heat the oil in a large non-stick pan and fry the onion over a low heat for 10 mins, stirring regularly, until softened and very lightly browned – add the garlic for the final min. Stir in the curry powder and cook for 30 secs more.

2 Add the lentils, 1 tsp flaked sea salt and 1 litre/1¾ pints of water. Stir in the sweet potatoes and bring to the boil. Reduce the heat to a simmer and cook the lentils for 50 mins or until the dhal is thick, stirring regularly. Add a splash of water if the dhal thickens too much. Stir in the lime or lemon juice and season to taste.

3 While the dhal is cooking, make the curried vegetables. Half-fill a medium non-stick pan with water and bring to the boil. Add the beans, cauliflower and carrots, and return to the boil. Cook for 4 mins, then drain.

4 Return the pan to the heat and add the oil and onion. Cook over a medium-high heat for 3-4 mins or until the onion is lightly browned, stirring regularly. Add the garlic and cook for 1 min more until softened. Stir in the curry powder and cook for a few secs, stirring.

5 Add the tomatoes, green chilli according to taste and 200ml/7fl oz cold water. Cook for 5 mins or until the tomatoes are well softened, stirring regularly. Stir in the blanched vegetables and cook for 4-5 mins or until hot throughout. Season with black pepper.

6 Divide the dhal among 4 deep bowls and top with the curried vegetables. Serve with the yogurt, coriander, green chilli slices and lime wedges for squeezing over.

TIP Freeze the dhal and vegetables in lidded freezer-proof containers for up to 3 months. Thaw overnight then add a splash of water and reheat until piping hot throughout.

BENEFITS vegetarian • low cal • low fat • iron • vit C • fibre • 5 of 5 a day
PER SERVING 453 kcals • fat 9g • saturates 1g • carbs 67g • sugars 23g • fibre 14g • protein 19g • salt 1.3g

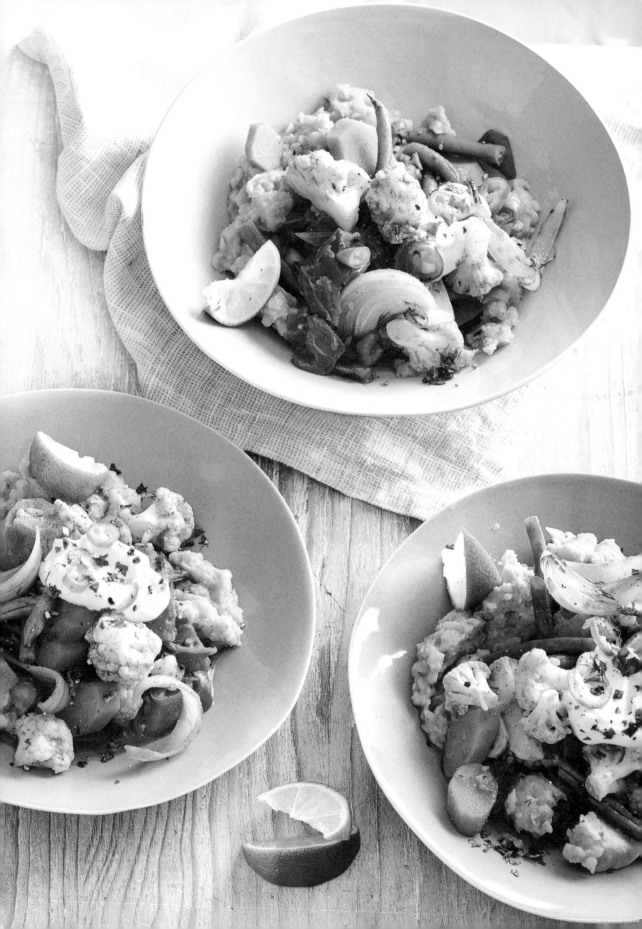

One-pot Chicken with Quinoa

An easy dish packed with vitamin-rich veg and mineral and protein rich quinoa
When cooking quinoa remember to rinse well and to cook until all the cooking water has been absorbed.

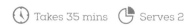 Takes 35 mins   Serves 2

- 1 tbsp rapeseed oil
- 2 skinless chicken breasts (about 300g/11oz)
- 1 medium onion, sliced into 12 wedges
- 1 red pepper, deseeded and sliced
- 2 garlic cloves, finely chopped
- 100g/4oz green beans, trimmed and cut in half
- ¼-½ tsp chilli flakes, according to taste
- 2 tsp each ground cumin and ground coriander
- 100g/4oz quinoa
- 85g/3oz frozen sweetcorn
- 75g/2½oz kale, thickly shredded

1 Heat the oil in a large, deep frying pan or sauté pan. Season the chicken and fry over a medium-high heat for 2-3 mins each side or until golden. Transfer to a plate. Add the onion and pepper to the pan and cook for 3 mins, stirring, until softened and lightly browned.

2 Tip in the garlic and beans, and stir-fry for 2 mins. Add the chilli and spices, then stir in the quinoa and sweetcorn. Pour in 700ml/1¼ pints just-boiled water and bring to the boil.

3 Return the chicken to the pan, reduce the heat to a simmer and cook for 12 mins, stirring regularly and turning the chicken occasionally. Add the kale and cook for a further 3 mins or until the quinoa and the chicken are cooked through.

BENEFITS low fat • folate • fibre • vit c • iron • 3 of 5 a day • gluten free
PER SERVING 529 kcals • fat 12g • saturates 1g • carbs 52g • sugars 15g • fibre 6g • protein 50g • salt 0.4g

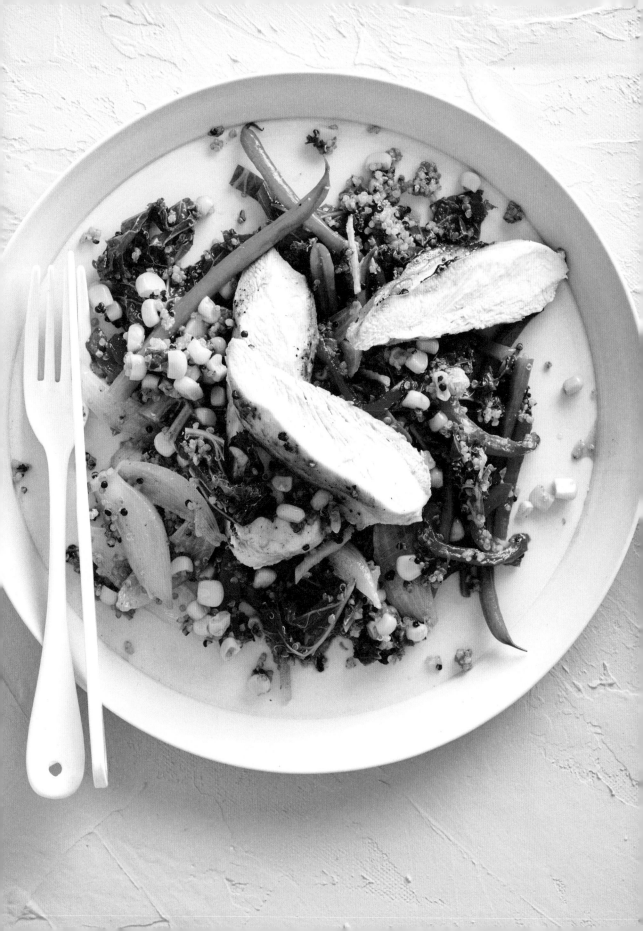

Steak & Sweet Potato Chips

This makes a great Friday night supper – satisfying and full of flavour yet immune-friendly, being rich in vitamin C and iron as well as beta-carotene.

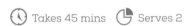 Takes 45 mins   Serves 2

- 350g/12oz sweet potatoes, peeled and cut into thick chips
- 1 tbsp rapeseed oil
- 2 x 200g/7oz sirloin steaks
- 50g bag mixed spinach, watercress & rocket salad
- 2 ripe tomatoes, cut into wedges
- ⅓ cucumber, sliced
- 2 spring onions, trimmed and finely sliced
- ½ x 400g can haricot beans, drained and rinsed

FOR THE DRESSING
- 2 tsp balsamic vinegar
- 2 tbsp rapeseed oil
- ½ small garlic clove, crushed

1 Heat oven to 220C/200C fan/gas 7. Half-fill a medium saucepan with water and bring to the boil. Add the sweet potatoes and cook for 4 mins, then drain through a colander and return to the saucepan. Pour over 2 tsp of the oil and season with a little black pepper. Toss until the potatoes are lightly coated with the oil.

2 Tip the potatoes onto a baking tray and cook in the oven for 15 mins, then turn with a spatula and cook for a further 10 mins or until crisp and golden.

3 While the potatoes are baking, prepare the steak. Trim off any hard fat from the beef, then rub all over with the remaining oil. Season with 1 tsp coarsely ground black pepper. Put a large non-stick frying pan or griddle over a medium-high heat and, when hot, add the steaks and cook for about 2 mins each side or until they are done to your liking.

4 Mix the salad leaves, tomatoes, cucumber, spring onions and beans in a bowl. Whisk the vinegar, oil and garlic together. Divide the steak, chips and salad between two plates and pour over the dressing just before serving.

BENEFITS *fibre • vit c • iron • 4 of 5 a day • gluten free*
PER SERVING *683 kcals • fat 29g • saturates 6g • carbs 49g • sugars 25g • fibre 13g • protein 48g • salt 0.6g*

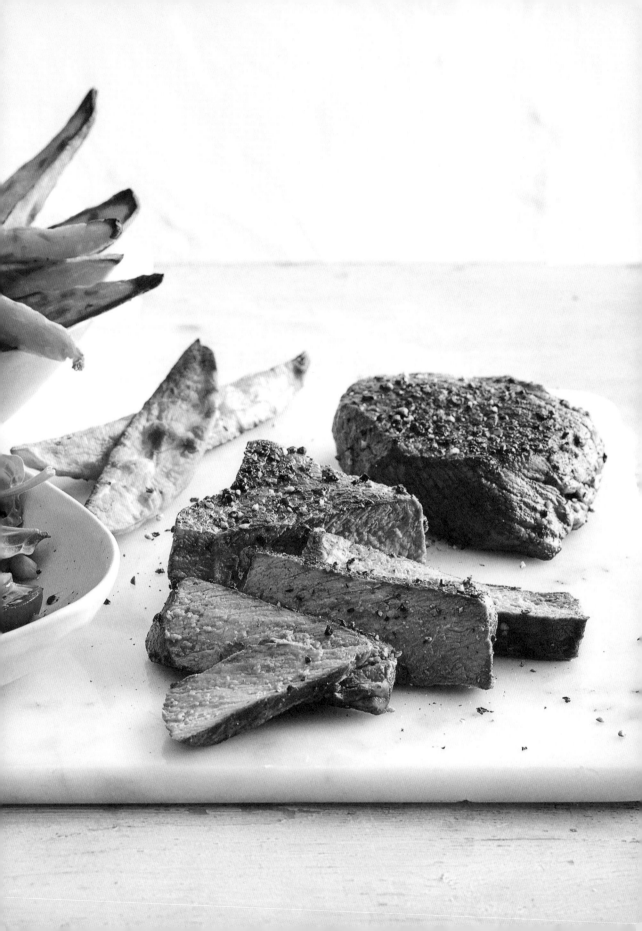

Lamb Dopiaza with Broccoli Rice

Simple and delicious, this low-fat curry is full of good things to nourish you – lean lamb, prebiotic onions and fibre-rich lentils.

🕐 Takes 1 hour 50 mins 🍽 Serves 4

- 500g/1lb 2oz lamb leg steaks, trimmed of excess fat and cut into chunks
- 100g/4oz bio live yogurt, plus 4 tbsp to serve
- 2 tbsp medium curry powder
- 2 tsp rapeseed oil
- 3 large onions, 2 thinly sliced, 1 cut into 10 wedges
- 4 garlic cloves, finely sliced
- 1 tbsp ginger, peeled and finely chopped
- 1 long red chilli, finely chopped (deseeded if you don't like it too hot)
- 400g/14oz tomatoes, roughly chopped or 400g can chopped tomatoes
- 100g/4oz dried red lentils, rinsed
- ½ small pack coriander, roughly chopped, plus extra to garnish
- 200g pack baby spinach leaves

FOR THE BROCCOLI RICE
- 200g/7oz brown basmati rice
- 200g/7oz small broccoli florets

1 Put the lamb in a large bowl and season well with ground black pepper. Add the yogurt and 1 tbsp of the curry powder, and stir well to combine.

2 Heat half the oil in a large non-stick saucepan. Fry the onion wedges over a high heat for 4-5 mins or until lightly browned and just tender. Tip onto a plate, set aside and return the pan to the heat.

3 Add the remaining oil, the sliced onions, garlic, ginger and chilli, cover and cook for 10 mins or until very soft, stirring occasionally. Remove the lid, increase the heat and cook for 2-3 mins more or until the onions are tinged with brown – this will add lots of flavour, but make sure they don't get burnt.

4 Reduce the heat once more and stir in the tomatoes and remaining curry powder. Cook for 1 min, then stir the lamb and yogurt into the pan and cook over a medium-high heat for 4-5 mins, stirring regularly.

5 Pour 250ml/9fl oz cold water into the pan, stir in the lentils and coriander, cover with a lid and leave to cook over a low heat for 45 mins – the sauce should be simmering gently. Remove the lid every 10-15 mins and stir the curry.

6 With half an hour of the curry cooking time remaining, cook the rice in plenty of boiling water for 25 mins or until just tender. Add the broccoli florets and cook for a further 3 mins. Drain well.

7 Remove the lid from the curry, add the reserved onion wedges and continue to simmer over a high heat for a further 15 mins or until the lamb is tender, stirring regularly. Just before serving, stir in the spinach, a handful at a time, and let it wilt. Serve with the yogurt, coriander and broccoli rice.

TIP You can freeze the cooked and cooled curry for up to 2 months. Thaw overnight in the fridge and reheat in a saucepan until piping hot throughout.

BENEFITS low fat • folate • fibre • vit c • iron • calcium • 4 of 5 a day
PER SERVING 620 kcals • fat 15g • saturates 5g • carbs 72g • sugars 17g • fibre 11g • protein 43g • salt 0.3g

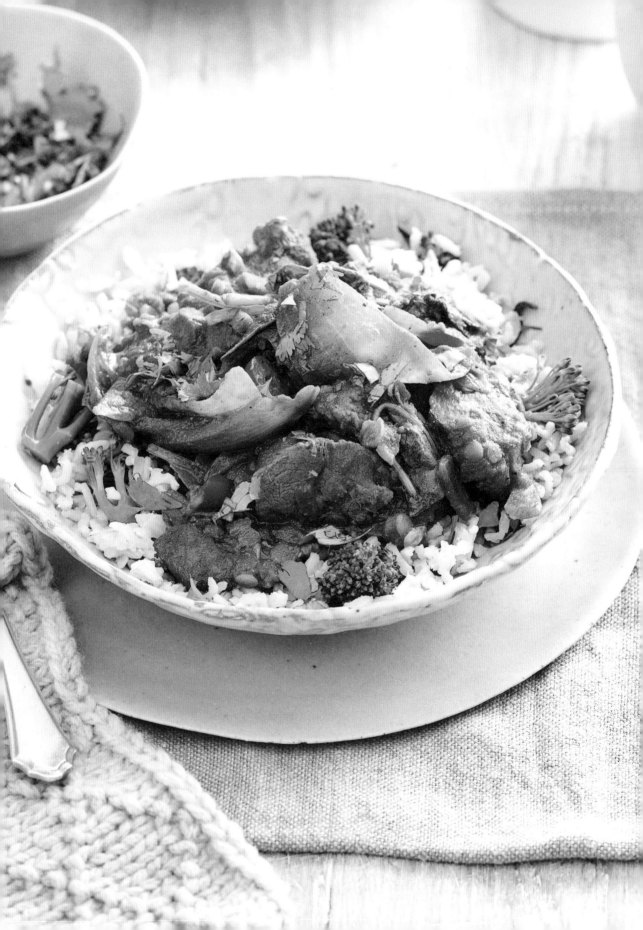

Cauliflower Crust Pizza

This is a bread-free, gluten-free pizza as cauliflower and ground almonds are used to make the base. Grind your own almonds with their skins on because flavonoids found in them more than doubles vitamin E's protective potency.

 Takes 30 mins Serves 4

- FOR THE BASE
- 1 cauliflower (about 750g/1lb 10oz)
- 100g/4oz ground almonds
- 2 eggs, beaten
- 1 tbsp dried oregano

FOR THE TOPPING
- ½ large aubergine, thinly sliced lengthways into long strips
- 2 tbsp olive oil, plus extra for greasing
- 1 small red onion, cut into 8 wedges
- 227g can chopped tomatoes
- 1 tbsp tomato purée
- 1 garlic clove, crushed
- the leaves from ½ small bunch basil
- 125g ball mozzarella
- 25g/1oz Parmesan or veggie alternative, grated, plus extra to serve
- a few pinches of chilli flakes

1 Heat oven to 200C/180C fan/gas 6. Remove the leaves from the cauliflower and trim the stalk end, then cut into chunks. Blitz half the cauliflower in a food processor until finely chopped, like rice. Transfer to a bowl and repeat with the remaining half. Tip all the cauliflower in a bowl, cover with cling film and microwave on High for 5-6 mins until softened. Tip onto a clean tea towel and leave to cool a little. Once cool enough to handle, scrunch up the tea towel and squeeze as much liquid as you can out of the cauliflower, then transfer to a clean bowl. Stir in the ground almonds, egg, oregano and plenty of seasoning. Line a baking tray with baking parchment and grease with oil. Mound the cauliflower mix into the centre of the tray, then use a spoon and your hands to spread out into a 30cm/12in round. Make it a little thicker at the edges to create a 'crust'. Bake for 15-18 mins until golden brown and starting to crisp a little at the edges.

2 Meanwhile, heat a griddle pan, brush each aubergine slice on both sides with a little of the oil, season and cook for 5-6 mins, turning once, until softened and charred – you'll need to do this in batches. Transfer to a plate. Brush the onions with oil, season and griddle for 5-8 mins until softened and charred. To make the tomato sauce, whizz the canned tomatoes, tomato purée, garlic and some seasoning in a blender until smooth. Transfer to a small saucepan, bring to a simmer and cook gently for 8-10 mins until thick (you don't want any watery tomato soaking into the cauliflower base). Tear half the basil leaves and stir through the sauce.

3 Once the cauliflower base is cooked, set aside to cool a little. Turn the oven up to 240C/220C fan/gas 8. Drain the mozzarella and pat dry with kitchen paper. Spread the tomato sauce over the base, sprinkle over the Parmesan, then arrange the aubergines, red onion and mozzarella on top. Scatter over the chilli flakes and return to the oven for 10-12 mins. Before serving, shave over a little more cheese and scatter with the remaining basil leaves.

BENEFITS vegetarian • fibre • 3 of 5 a day • gluten free
PER SERVING 436 kcals • fat 33g • saturates 9g • carbs 12g • sugars 12g • fibre 8g • protein 26g • salt 0.7g

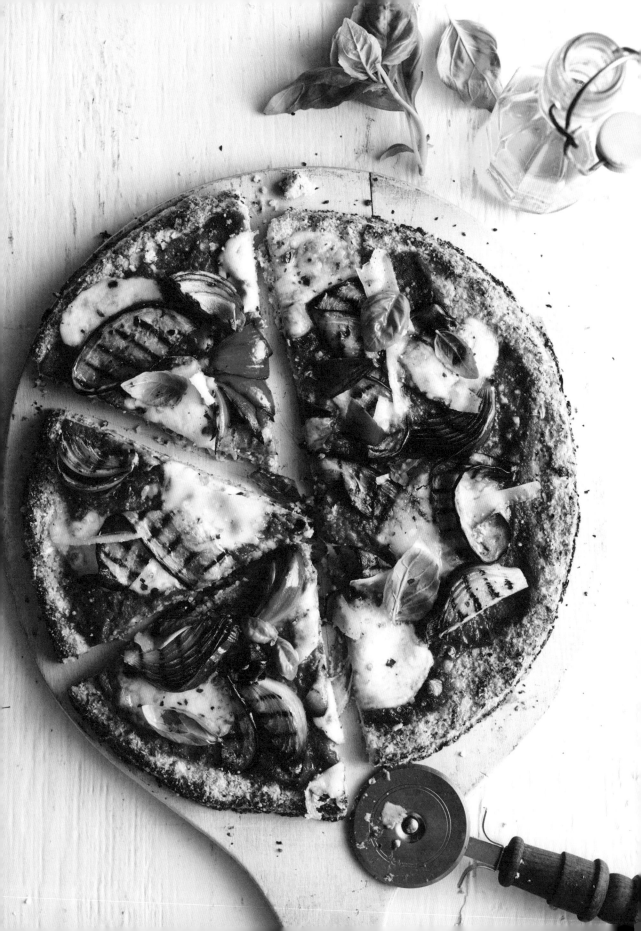

Squash,
Mushroom & Gorgonzola Pilaf

This is deliciously savoury and filling, and surprisingly low in calories as a little strong flavoured cheese goes a long way.

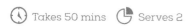 Takes 50 mins   Serves 2

- 1 tsp rapeseed oil
- 1 large onion, halved and sliced
- 3 garlic cloves, finely chopped
- 200g/7oz chunk butternut squash, peeled, deseeded and diced
- 140g/5oz button mushrooms, halved if large
- 125g/4½oz brown basmati rice
- 700ml/1¼ pints reduced-salt vegetable bouillion
- 10 pieces dried mushrooms, chopped
- 2 tsp chopped sage leaves
- small pack parsley leaves and stalks separated, chopped
- 40g/1½oz gorgonzola, crumbled

1 Heat the oil in a large non-stick pan, add the onion and garlic, and fry for 5 mins. Tip in the squash and mushrooms, and cook a few mins more. Stir in the rice, then pour in the stock. Stir well, then add the dried mushrooms, sage and parsley stalks. Cover and simmer over a low heat for 35–40 mins until the rice is tender. Check towards the end of cooking and add a little water if the rice has absorbed all the stock.

2 Remove from the heat, fold in the parsley leaves and the cheese with a grinding of black pepper, then allow to stand for 5 mins before serving.

BENEFITS vegetarian • low fat • low cal • fibre • vit c • 3 of 5 a day
PER SERVING 422 kcals • fat 10g • saturates 5g • carbs 63g • sugars 13g • fibre 10g • protein 17g • salt 0.9g

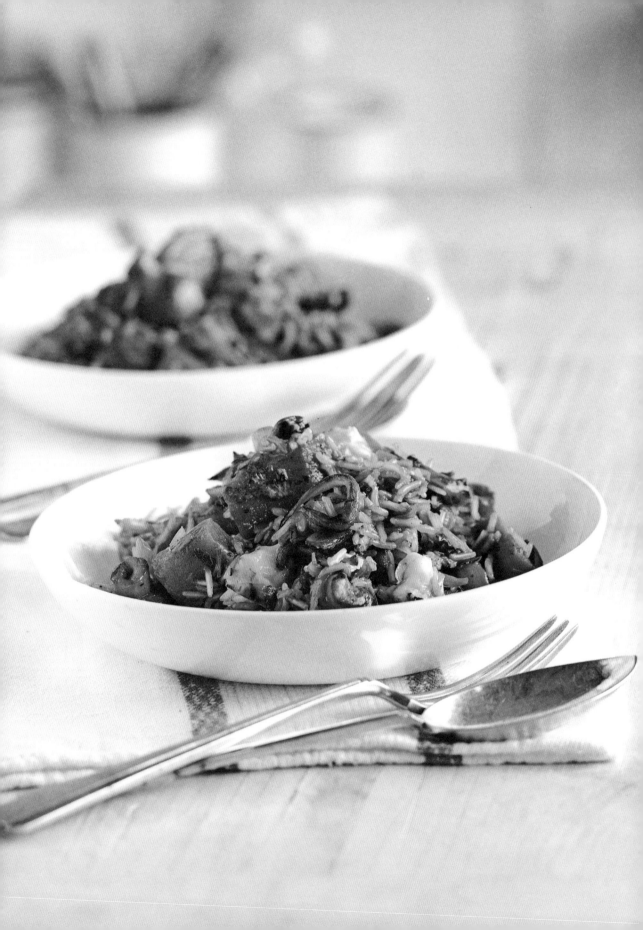

Light Thai Green Curry

Thai curries can be quite high in fat so we've reduced the fat by mixing oat milk with a small amount of creamed coconut. You can use the green curry paste for other recipes too.

🕐 TAKES 1 hour 20 mins   ◔ Serves 2

- 25g/1oz rolled oats, soaked in 200ml/7fl oz cold water for 20 mins
- 1½ tbsp creamed coconut, grated
- 1 tsp coconut oil or rapeseed oil
- 2 carrots, sliced
- 1 parsnip, cut into small chunks
- 1 small sweet potato, chopped into small pieces
- 2 kaffir lime leaves (dried or fresh)
- 6 spears purple sprouting broccoli, halved lengthways
- 50g/2oz frozen peas
- 1 lime, cut into 6 wedges

FOR THE GREEN CURRY PASTE
- 1 green pepper, deseeded and chopped
- ½ small pack coriander
- 1 garlic clove, peeled
- 2cm/¾in piece of ginger,
- peeled zest and juice 1 lime
- 2 spring onions, roughly chopped
- 1 green chilli, deseeded and roughly chopped

TO SERVE
- brown basmati rice
- ½ small pack coriander (optional)

1 First, make the curry paste. Put all the ingredients in the small bowl of a food processor and blitz until finely chopped. Transfer to a small bowl and chill.

2 Put the oats and their soaking water in the food processor (no need to clean it first) and blend until it's as smooth as you can get it. Strain it through a sieve to get rid of any remaining oats, then add the creamed coconut and set aside.

3 Put a large, non-stick frying pan or wok over a high heat. Add the coconut oil followed by the carrot, parsnip and sweet potato. Stir-fry for about 2-3 mins until the vegetables start to colour at the edges, then add the curry paste and cook until the curry no longer looks watery. Pour in the oat milk and coconut mixture, lime leaves and 300ml/½ pint water, and bring to a simmer. Cover and cook for 15 mins, then add the broccoli, along with 50ml/2fl oz water and cook for 5 mins more or until tender. Finally, add the frozen peas for 1 min more or until hot through. Take the pan off the heat, then squeeze over the juice from 2 of the lime wedges.

4 Serve immediately with brown rice, the remaining lime wedges and a scattering of coriander leaves, if you like.

BENEFITS vegetarian • low fat • calcium • folate • fibre • vit c • iron • 5 of 5 a day
PER SERVING 434 kcals • fat 14g • saturates 2g • carbs 54g • sugars 21g • fibre 21g • protein 11g • salt 0.2g

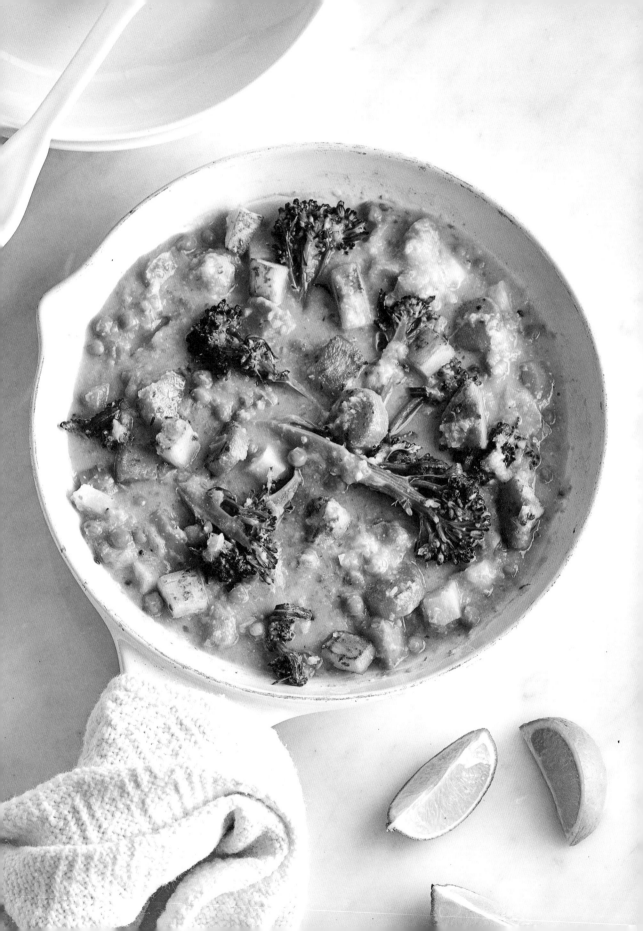

Meatballs with Fennel & Balsamic Beans & Courgette Noodles

Rich in immune-friendly nutrients like vitamin C and beta-carotene, courgettes are used instead of pasta here as a delicious gluten-free alternative. Courgettes are high in water content, so filling yet low in calories.

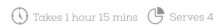 Takes 1 hour 15 mins Serves 4

- 400g pack lean steak mince
- 2 tsp dried oregano
- 1 large egg
- 8 garlic cloves, 1 finely grated, the others sliced
- 1-2 tbsp rapeseed oil
- 1 fennel bulb, finely chopped, fronds reserved
- 2 carrots, finely chopped
- 500g carton passata
- 4 tbsp balsamic vinegar
- 600ml/1 pint reduced-salt vegetable bouillon

FOR THE COURGETTE NOODLES
- 1 tsp rapeseed oil
- 1-2 large courgettes, cut into noodles with a julienne peeler or spiralizer
- 300g/11oz frozen soya beans, thawed

1. Put the mince, oregano, egg and grated garlic in a bowl and grind in some black pepper. Mix together thoroughly and roll into 16 balls.
2. Heat the oil in a large sauté pan over a medium-high heat, add the meatballs and fry, moving them around the pan so that they brown all over – be careful as they're quite delicate and you don't want them to break up. Once brown, remove them from the pan. Reduce the heat slightly and add the fennel, carrots and sliced garlic to the pan and fry, stirring until they soften, about 5 mins.
3. Tip in the passata, balsamic vinegar and bouillon, stir well, then return the meatballs to the pan, cover and cook gently for 20-25 mins.
4. Meanwhile, heat the 1 tsp of oil in a non-stick pan and stir-fry the courgette with the beans to heat through and soften. Serve with the meatballs and scatter with any fennel fronds. The meatballs will keep in the fridge for a couple of days or freeze.

BENEFITS low fat • low cal • folate • fibre • vit c • iron • 4 of 5 a day
PER SERVING 380 kcals • fat 14g • saturates 3g • carbs 20g • sugars 15g • fibre 11g • protein 37g •
salt 0.5g

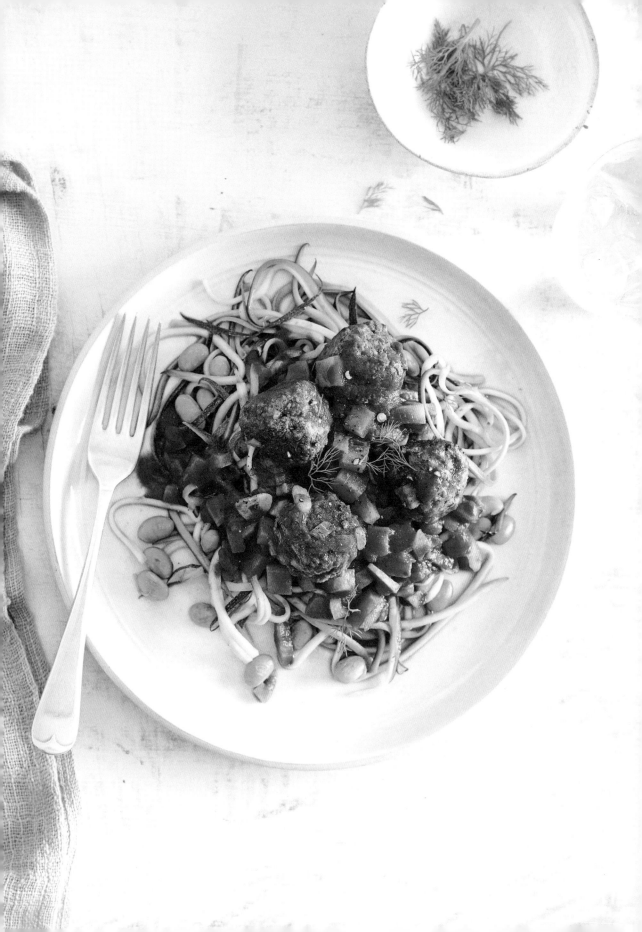

Zingy Teriyaki Beef Skewers

This is flavoured with ginger, which protects and heals the gut and eases stomach upsets and nausea. The brown rice, a whole grain, is rich in minerals including zinc

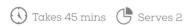 Takes 45 mins   Serves 2

- 1 tbsp wheat-free tamari
- 3 tbsp freshly squeezed orange juice
- 15g/½oz chunk of ginger, peeled and very finely grated
- 2 garlic cloves, crushed
- 1 tsp honey (preferably raw)
- ¼ tsp chilli flakes
- 300g/11oz beef sirloin steak, trimmed of hard fat and cut into long, thin strips

FOR THE SALAD
- 100g/4oz brown basmati rice
- ⅓ cucumber, cut into small cubes
- 2 carrots, peeled and sliced into ribbons with a peeler
- 4 spring onions, trimmed and diagonally sliced
- 100g/4oz radishes, trimmed and sliced
- small pack coriander, leaves roughly chopped, plus extra to garnish
- handful mint leaves, plus extra to garnish
- 1 tbsp rapeseed oil
- zest and juice 1 lime
- 25g/1oz unsalted cashew nuts, toasted and roughly chopped

1 Put the tamari, orange juice, ginger, garlic, honey and chilli flakes in a small saucepan with 100ml/3½fl oz cold water and bring to the boil. Cook for 3-5 mins, boiling hard until well reduced, glossy and slightly syrupy. Remove from the heat, pour into a shallow dish and leave to cool.

2 Thread the beef onto 4 soaked wooden or metal skewers. Place in the marinade, turn and brush until well coated. Cover with cling film and marinate for 30 mins.

3 While the beef is marinating, prepare the salad. Half-fill a medium pan with water and bring to the boil. Cook the rice for about 20 mins or following pack instructions until tender. Rinse in a sieve under running water until cold, then drain well. Tip into a large bowl.

4 Add the cucumber, carrots, spring onions, radishes, coriander, mint, oil, lime zest and juice, and toss together well. Season with a little black pepper. Divide between 2 plates and top with a sprinkling of nuts and extra herbs to garnish.

5 Heat the grill to high. (You could also cook the skewers on a non-stick griddle pan.) Put the skewers on a rack above a foil-lined baking tray, reserving any excess marinade. Grill the skewers close to the heat for 3-5 mins each side or until done to your liking. Brush with more marinade when they are turned. They should look sticky and glossy when cooked. Serve hot or cold with the rice salad.

BENEFITS folate • fibre•vit c•iron•3 of 5 a day • gluten fr
PER SERVING 563 kcals • fat 22g • saturates 6g • carbs 46g • sugars 16g • fibre 9g • protein 39g • salt 1.4g

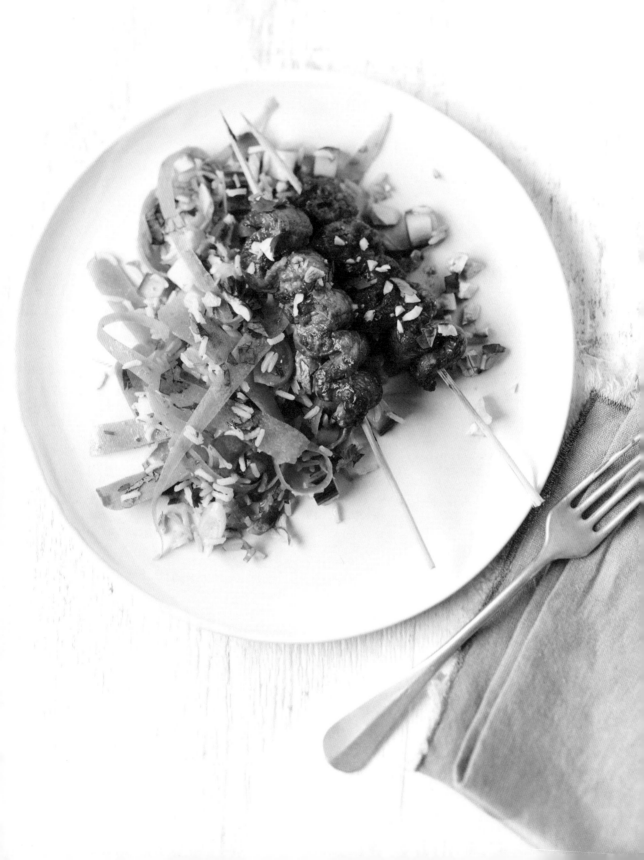

Chicken Katsu Curry

This katsu is coated in finely chopped flaked almonds and baked in the oven (rather than fried) until crisp and golden.

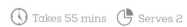 Takes 55 mins   Serves 2

- 25g/1oz flaked almonds
- 1 tsp rapeseed oil
- 2 small boneless, skinless chicken breasts (about 300g/11oz total)
- lime wedges, for serving

FOR THE SAUCE
- 2 tsp rapeseed oil
- 1 onion, roughly chopped
- 2 garlic cloves, finely chopped
- thumb-sized piece of ginger, peeled and finely chopped
- 2 tsp medium curry powder
- 1 star anise
- ¼ tsp ground turmeric
- 1 tbsp wholemeal flour

FOR THE RICE
- 100g/4oz brown basmati rice
- 2 spring onions, finely sliced (include the green part)

FOR THE SALAD
- 1 carrot, peeled into strips with a vegetable peeler
- ⅓ cucumber, peeled into strips with a vegetable peeler
- 1 small red chilli, finely chopped (deseeded if you don't like it too hot)
- juice ½ lime
- small handful each mint and coriander leaves

1 Heat oven to 220C/200C fan/gas 7. Cook the brown rice in plenty of boiling water for 35 mins or until very tender.

2 Crush the almonds using a pestle and mortar, or blitz in a food processor until finely chopped, then sprinkle over a plate. Grease a small baking tray with a little of the oil. Brush the chicken on both sides with the remaining oil and season well. Coat the chicken with the nuts and place on the tray. Press any remaining nuts from the plate onto each breast. Bake for 20 mins or until browned and cooked through. Rest for 4-5 mins on the tray, then slice the chicken thickly.

3 Meanwhile, make the sauce. Heat the oil in a medium non-stick saucepan and add the onion, garlic and ginger. Loosely cover the pan and fry gently for 8 mins or until softened and lightly browned, stirring occasionally. Remove the lid for the final 2 mins, and don't let the garlic burn.

4 Stir in the curry powder, star anise, turmeric and a good grinding of black pepper. Cook for a few secs more, stirring. Sprinkle over the flour and stir well. Gradually add 400ml/14fl oz water to the pan, stirring constantly.

5 Bring the sauce to a simmer and cook for 10 mins, stirring occasionally. If it begins to splutter, cover loosely with a lid. Remove the pan from the heat and blitz the sauce with a stick blender until very smooth. Adjust the seasoning to taste. Keep warm.

6 Once the rice is tender, add the spring onions and cook for 1 min more. Drain well, then leave to stand for a few mins while you make the salad. Toss the carrot and cucumber with the chilli, lime juice and herbs.

7 Divide the sliced chicken between 2 plates, pour over the sauce and serve with the rice, salad and lime wedges for squeezing over.

BENEFITS fibre • iron • 2 of 5 a day
PER SERVING 585 kcals • fat 16g • saturates 2g • carbs 58g • sugars 12g • fibre 9g • protein 47g • salt 0.3g

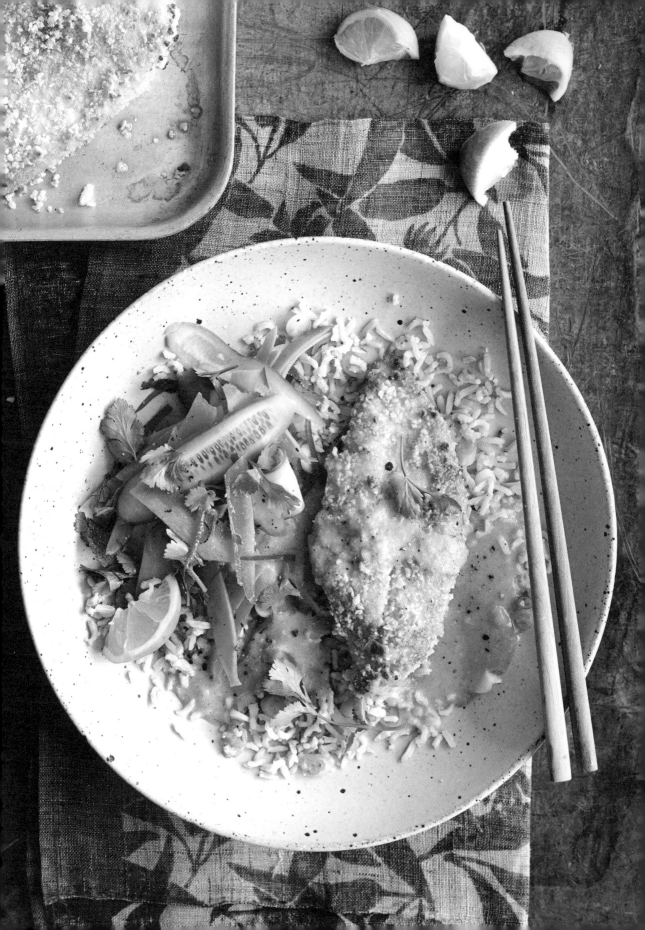

Zesty Salmon with Roasted Beets & Spinach

Experts tell us to eat a rainbow of different coloured fruit and veg so we benefit from a wide range of nutrients and phyto-chemicals. We've packed in as many as we can in this delicious salad - green avocado and spinach, fresh oranges and deep purple beets.

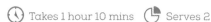 Takes 1 hour 10 mins   Serves 2

- 4 small fresh beetroots (about 200g/7oz)
- 1½ tbsp cold-pressed rapeseed oil
- 1 tsp coriander seeds, lightly crushed
- 2 skinless salmon (preferably wild) or trout fillets
- 2½ small oranges, zest of 1, juice of ½
- 3 tbsp pumpkin seeds
- 1 garlic clove
- 1 red onion, finely chopped
- 4 handfuls baby spinach leaves
- 1 avocado, stoned, peeled and thickly sliced

1 Heat oven to 180C/160C fan/gas 4. Trim the stems of the beetroots and reserve any tender leaves that are suitable for eating in the salad. Quarter the beetroots, then toss with ½ tbsp oil, the coriander seeds and some seasoning. Pile onto the centre of a large sheet of foil and wrap up into a parcel. Bake for 45 mins or until the beetroots are tender, then top with the salmon, scatter over the zest of half an orange and wrap up once more, returning to the oven for 15 mins. If you want to toast the pumpkin seeds, put them in the oven for 10 mins.

2 Meanwhile, cut the peel and pith from 2 oranges, then cut out the segments with a sharp knife, working over a bowl to catch the juices. Finely grate the garlic and leave for 10 mins to allow the enzymes to activate. Stir the garlic into the orange juice and remaining oil, with seasoning, to make a dressing.

3 Remove the parcel from the oven and lift out the fish. Tip the beetroot into a bowl with the red onion, zest of half an orange, the pumpkin seeds and spinach, and mix well. Gently toss through the orange segments and avocado with any beet leaves, then pile onto plates and top with the warm salmon. Drizzle over the dressing and serve while still warm.

BENEFITS calcium • folate • fibre • vit c • iron • omega 3 • 4 of 5 a day • gluten free
PER SERVING 543 kcals • fat 32g • saturates 5g • carbs 27g • sugars 22g • fibre 10g • protein 33g • salt 0.6g

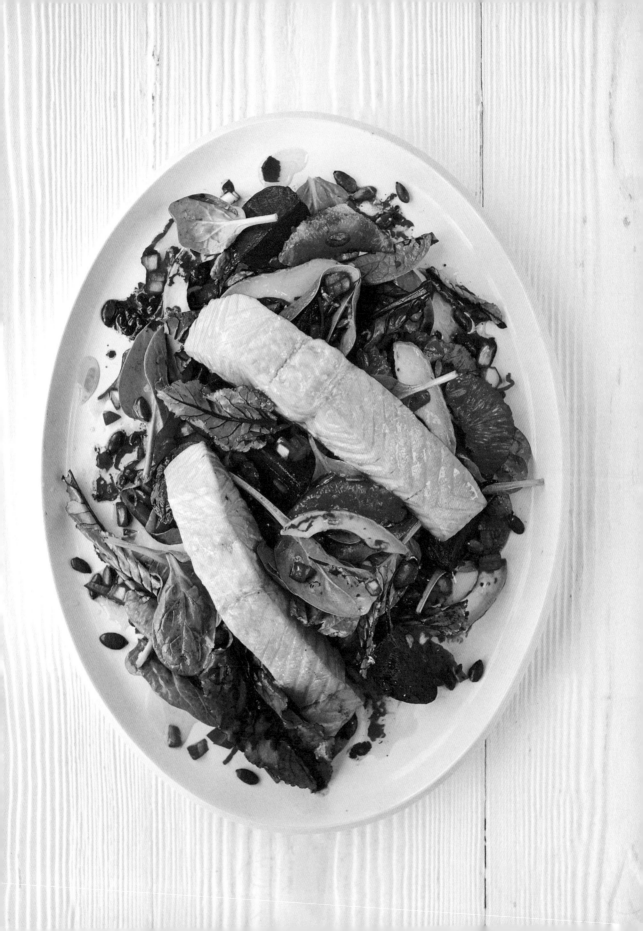

Trout with Tomato Sauce

Serve this oily fish supper with steamed veg like broccoli or wilted spinach with brown rice or new potatoes cooked in their skins.

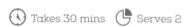 Takes 30 mins Serves 2

- 1½ tbsp olive oil
- 1 shallot, thinly sliced
- 2 garlic cloves, crushed
- 1 bay leaf
- 400g can chopped tomatoes
- 1 tsp apple cider vinegar
- 1 tbsp butter
- 2 rainbow trout fillets, pin-boned, skin left on (if the fillets are large, cut in half lengthways or ask your fishmonger to do this for you)
- handful mixed olives, stones removed
- handful basil, shredded
- extra virgin olive oil, for drizzling

1 In a frying pan, heat 1 tbsp of oil over a low-medium heat. Add the shallot and a pinch of salt, then cook, stirring occasionally, for 8 mins until softened and the edges begin to brown. Stir in the garlic and cook for 1 min, then add the bay leaf, tomatoes, vinegar and seasoning. Stir well, bring to the boil, then reduce the heat and simmer gently for 15 mins.

2 After the sauce has been simmering for 7 mins, heat the remaining oil with the butter in a non-stick frying pan over a medium-high heat. Season the fish well and place, skin-side down, in the pan. Cook for 4 mins – try not to move the fish so the skin gets evenly coloured. Flip over and continue to cook for 2 mins or until the flesh begins to flake in large chunks.

3 Spoon some sauce onto each plate and top with a fillet. Scatter over the olives and the basil, then drizzle over the extra virgin olive oil to serve.

BENEFITS vit c • omega-3 • 1 of 5 a day • gluten free
PER SERVING 429 kcals • fat 25g • saturates 8g • carbs 9g • sugars 8g • fibre 2g • protein 40g • salt 0.9g

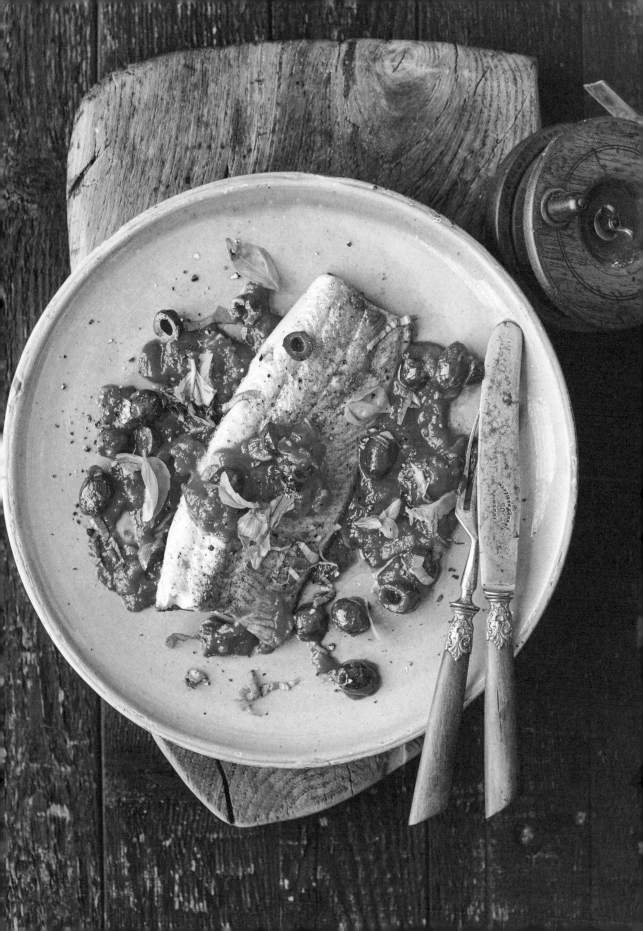

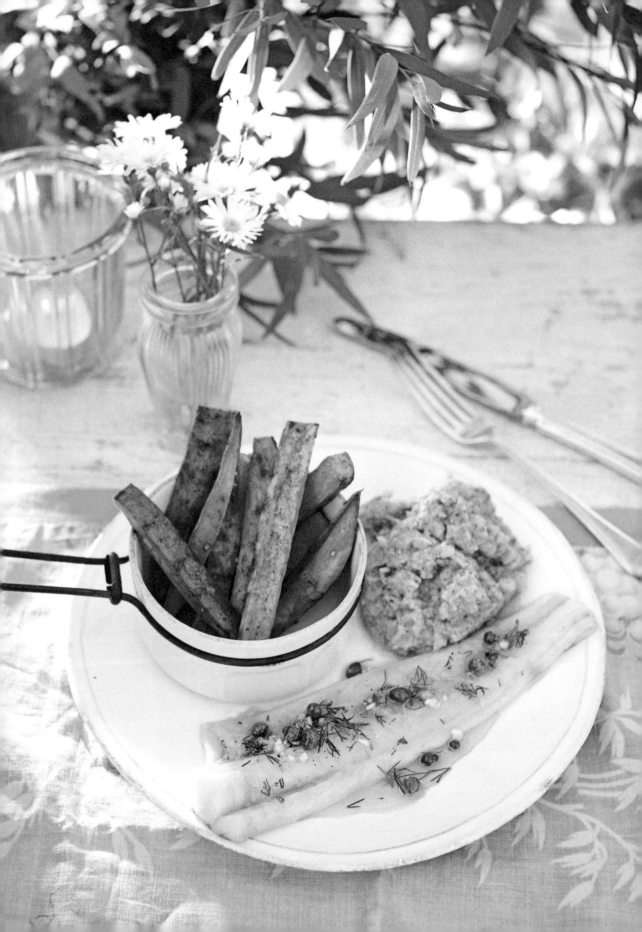

Chapter 2

THE 7-DAY VITALITY PLAN

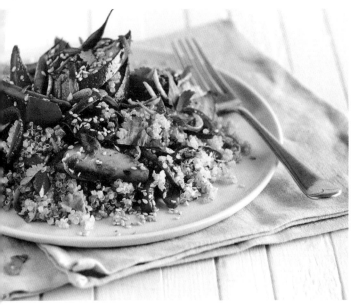

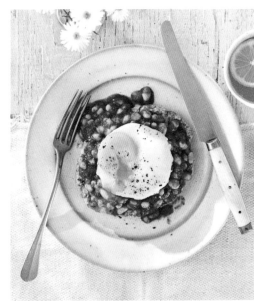

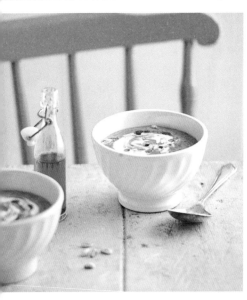

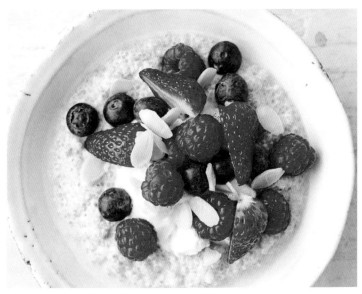

Eat to look & feel fabulous

The healthiest way to looking and feeling your absolute best is to follow a nutritious and balanced eating plan combined with some physical activity and relaxation.

How you look and feel can be influenced by a number of factors – stress, chemical overload, pollution, prolonged exposure to the sun, poor sleep and a diet of processed, sugary foods and alcohol all take their toll. By following an eating plan rich in healthy, natural fats, lean protein with a wide variety of fruits, vegetables, nuts, seeds and whole grains you can arm your body with the protection it needs to fend off the signs of aging.

Looking fabulous
We all want plump, youthful skin but as the largest organ of the body, our skin can be the first to show the signs of wear and tear. Vitamins including A, C and E are all vital for healthy, well-supported skin. We've included these nutrients from ingredients like sweet potato and squash, peppers and citrus as well as avocado.

Lean protein like fish, chicken, pulses and eggs are important to supply the building blocks needed for skin turnover and regeneration. We also need protein for healthy, lustrous hair and strong nails. Our plan ensures a consistent supply of protein throughout each day, unlike the typical western diet, which tends to be carb heavy at breakfast and lunch.

Although most of us have grown to fear the fat in our diets, our plan incorporates good fats in order to promote strong, moisturised skin. As we age our skin becomes thinner so it's important to ensure it remains a strong barrier to our environment – fat helps because our skin cells need the right types of fats for the formation of strong cell walls.

Feeling great
It's not just how we look that can affect how vital we feel. How fit and healthy our brains remain as we age is key to us feeling well and living life to the full. The right type of fat is essential for a well-functioning mind. That's why we've included oily fish like sardines and salmon as well as plant sources of these brain-friendly essential fats – the omega-3 fatty acids - from walnuts and almonds. Aim to include at least one portion of oily fish in your diet each week.

Our vitality plan is carefully balanced to supply slow-release carbs combined with protein to help keep you full and satisfied and your brain fuelled, preventing mood-changing blood sugar swings.

Fruit and vegetables are key to maintaining a sharp and active mind. Berries like blueberries are packed with protective compounds, called anthocyanins, which help the brain mop up damaged cells and so reduce the damage that contributes to cognitive decline. Green leafy veg supply the B vitamins, which studies suggest are important for brain health and aging.

Low levels of iron can lead to poor concentration as well as low energy and is a common problem among women and girls. We've included recipes in the vitality plan that contribute a third of your daily iron needs. Try to avoid drinking tea with your meals as this can block your iron absorption by up to 50%.

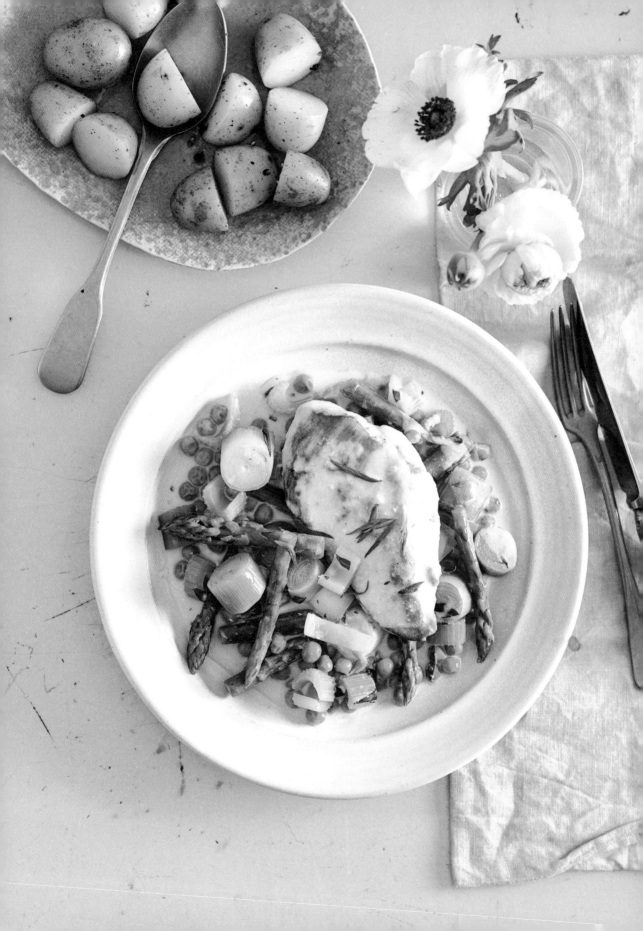

Once you've completed the 7 days you can start to build your own vitality plan using the additional recipes in this chapter – all our recipes are packed with key ingredients bursting with vitamins, minerals and phytonutrients as well as healthy fats and lean protein to keep you functioning at your optimal.

The secret to the success of any approach to healthy eating is preparation and planning, so we recommend using the Saturday before you start the plan to do the shopping as well as a little bit of food prep.

We suggest you enjoy the meals as set out in the 7-day vitality chart for the most nutritionally balanced approach, but if you do want to mix, match or repeat dishes, you'll still get all the benefits of eating unprocessed and wholesome foods.

THE 7-DAY VITALITY PLAN (Serves 2)

	BREAKFAST	LUNCH	DINNER
Sunday	Date & buckwheat granola with pecans & seeds	Barley couscous & prawn tabbouleh	Herby lamb fillet with caponata
Monday	Coconut quinoa & chia porridge	Summer pistou	Spicy vegetable pilau with cucumber raita
Tuesday	Date & buckwheat granola with pecans & seeds	Herb pancake wraps with goat's cheese	Roast chicken with sweet potato gremolata salad
Wednesday	Coconut quinoa & chia porridge	Summer pistou	Veggie meatballs with tomato courgetti
Thursday	Date & buckwheat granola with pecans & seeds	Peanut houmous with fruit & veg sticks	Chicken & avocado salad with blueberry dressing
Friday	Date & buckwheat granola with pecans & seeds	Asparagus & lentil salad with crumbled feta	Lemon pollock with sweet potato chips
Saturday	Wholemeal yogurt flatbreads with beans & poached egg	Peanut houmous with fruit & veg sticks	Salmon with corn & pepper salsa salad

Date & Buckwheat Granola with Pecans & Seeds

Granola is usually loaded with fat and sugar, but his version uses a date purée to sweeten the buckwheat as it cooks, which also encourages the ingredients to clump together into crunchy clusters.

 Takes 45 mins, plus overnight soaking   Serves 8

FOR THE GRANOLA
- 85g/3oz buckwheat
- 4 Medjool dates, stoned
- 1 tsp ground cinnamon
- 100g/4oz traditional oats
- 2 tsp rapeseed oil
- 25g/1oz each sunflower and pumpkin seeds
- 25g/1oz flaked almonds
- 50g/2oz pecan nuts, roughly broken into halves
- 50g/2oz sultanas

FOR THE YOGURT & FRUIT
(to serve 2)
- 2 x 150ml pots live bio yogurt
- 2 ripe nectarines or peaches, stoned and sliced

1 Soak the buckwheat overnight in cold water. The next day, drain and rinse the buckwheat. Put the dates in a pan with 300ml/½ pint water and the cinnamon, and blitz with a stick blender until completely smooth. Add the buckwheat, bring to the boil and cook, uncovered, for 5 mins until pulpy. Meanwhile, heat oven to 150C/130C fan/gas 2 and line 2 large baking trays with some baking parchment.

2 Stir the oats and oil into the date and buckwheat mixture, then spoon small clusters of the mixture onto the baking trays. Bake for 15 mins, then carefully scrape the clusters from the parchment if they have stuck and turn before spreading out again. Return to the oven for another 15 mins, turning frequently, until firm and golden.

3 When the mix is dry enough, tip into a bowl, mix in the seeds and nuts with the sultanas and toss well. When cool, serve each person a generous handful with yogurt and fruit, and pack the excess into an airtight container. Will keep for a week. On other days you can vary the fruit or serve with milk or a dairy-free alternative instead of the yogurt.

BENEFITS vegetarian • calcium • vit c • 1 of 5 a day
PER SERVING 421 kcals • fat 15g • saturates 4g • carbs 50g • sugars 34g • fibre 3g • protein 16g • salt 0.3g

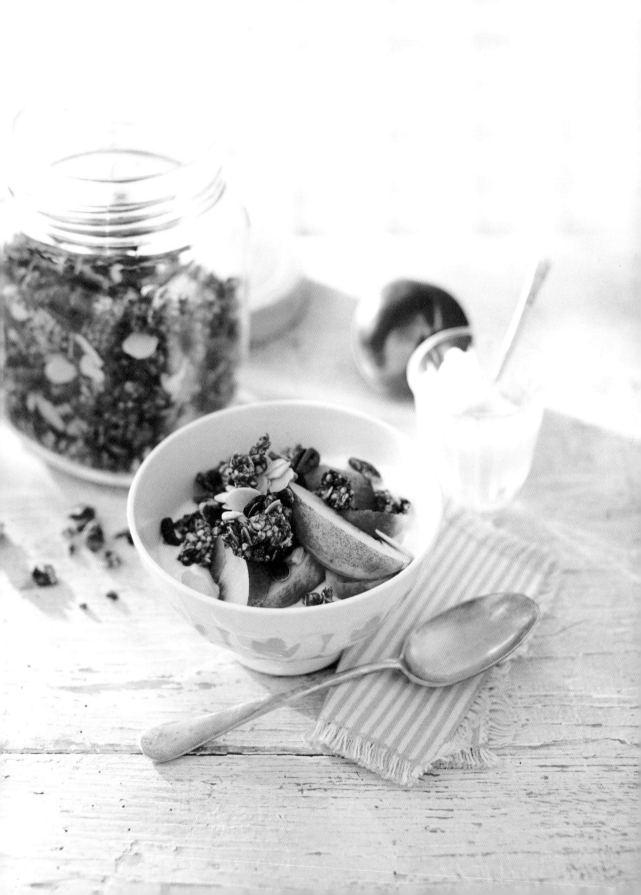

Coconut Quinoa & Chia Porridge with Berries & Almonds

This yummy porridge features high-protein quinoa and omega-3-rich chia seeds for a nutrient-packed breakfast topped with berries. Save time and make double if you like, as you will have it as part of the plan later in the week or see the recipe overleaf.

 Takes 35 mins, plus overnight soaking   Serves 2

FOR THE PORRIDGE
- 85g/3oz quinoa
- ¼ vanilla pod, split and seeds scraped out, or ¼tsp vanilla extract
- 7g/¼oz creamed coconut
- 2 tbsp chia seeds
- half a 125g pot coconut yogurt e.g. CoYo

FOR THE TOPPING
- half 125g pot coconut yogurt
- 280g/10oz mixed summer berries, such as strawberries, raspberries and blueberries
- 2 tbsp flaked almonds (optional)

1 Activate the quinoa by soaking overnight in cold water. The next day, drain and rinse the quinoa through a fine sieve (the grains are so small that they will wash through a coarse one).

2 Tip the quinoa into a pan and add the vanilla, creamed coconut and 600ml water. Cover the pan and simmer for 20 mins. Stir in the chia with another 300ml water and cook gently for 3 mins more. Stir in the half pot of coconut yogurt. Spoon half the porridge into a bowl for another day. Will keep for 2 days covered in the fridge. Serve the remaining porridge topped with remaining yogurt, the berries and almonds, if you like.

3 If making double to have the porridge another day, it will keep for 2 days covered in the fridge. To serve, tip the porridge into a pan and reheat gently, with milk or water then top with fruit.

TIP Blueberries are rich in protective anthocyanins, which are brain-friendly, helping to maintain memory and function.

BENEFITS *vegan • fibre • vit c • iron • omega-3 • 2 of 5 a day • gluten free*
PER SERVING 412 kcals • fat 21g • saturates 14g • carbs 36g • sugars 13g • fibre 12g • protein 12g • salt 0.1g

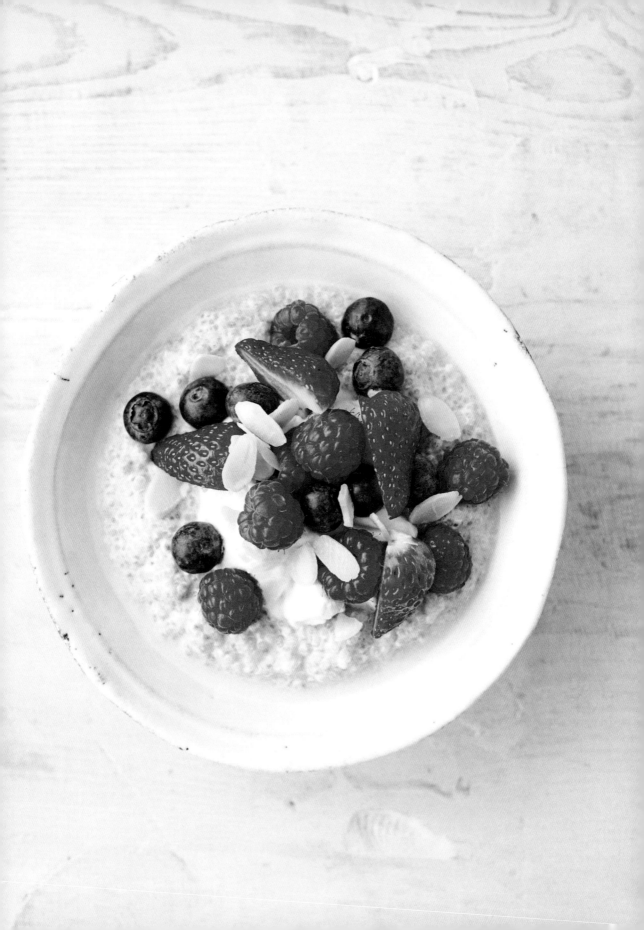

Quinoa & Chia Porridge with Oranges & Pomegranate Seeds

Vitamin C packed fresh oranges with crunchy pomegranate seeds make the zingy topping for this breakfast. Chop the oranges rather than segment them to include as much of their fibre as possible.

 Takes 35 mins, plus overnight soaking Serves 2

FOR THE PORRIDGE
- 85g/3oz quinoa
- ¼ vanilla pod, split and seeds scraped out, or ¼tsp vanilla extract or a generous sprinkle cinnamon
- 7g/¼oz creamed coconut
- 2 tbsp chia seeds
- half a 125g pot coconut yogurt e.g. CoYo

FOR THE TOPPING
- 2 oranges, peeled and chopped
- the seeds from ½ pomegranate

1 Activate the quinoa by soaking overnight in cold water. The next day, drain and rinse the quinoa through a fine sieve (the grains are so small that they will wash through a coarse one).

2 Tip the quinoa into a pan and add the vanilla or cinnamon, creamed coconut and 600ml water. Cover the pan and simmer for 20 mins. Stir in the chia with another 300ml water and cook gently for 3 mins more. Stir in the coconut yogurt. Spoon into bowls and top with the oranges and pomegranate seeds.

BENEFITS vegan • fibre • vit C • iron • omega 3 • 1 of 5 a day • gluten free
PER SERVING 350 kcals • fat 15g • saturates 8g • carbs 36g • sugars 14g • fibre 10g • protein 11g • salt 0.1g

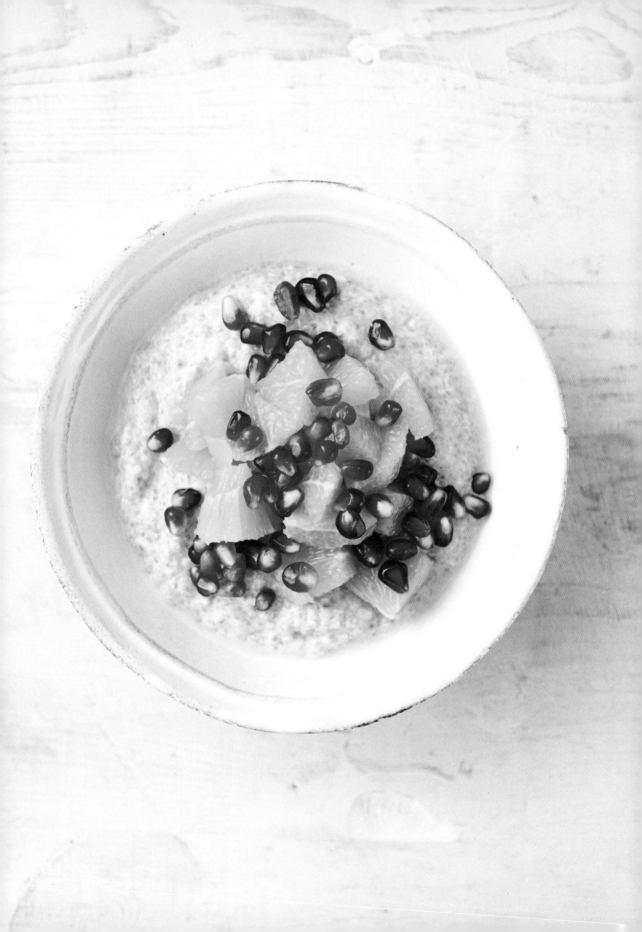

Wholemeal Yogurt Flatbreads with Beans & Poached Egg

This makes a really substantial brunch, so if you're eating earlier for breakfast, serve half the beans and keep the rest for another day.

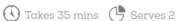 Takes 35 mins Serves 2

- 2 eggs

FOR THE BEANS
- 500g carton passata
- 2 small onions, quartered
- 1 Medjool date, stoned
- 3 tsp smoked paprika
- 1 tsp balsamic vinegar
- 400g can haricot beans, drained

FOR THE FLATBREADS
- 100g/4oz wholewheat flour
- ½ tsp baking powder
- 100g/4oz live bio yogurt

1 Tip the passata into a food processor with the onions, date and paprika, and blitz until completely smooth. Heat in a medium pan, cover and simmer for 10 mins, stirring frequently, to make a thick pulpy sauce. Taste to make sure the onion is fully cooked. If not, add a splash of water and cook a little longer. Stir in the vinegar and beans, then remove from the heat.

2 To make the flatbreads, tip the flour and baking powder into a bowl, then stir in the yogurt to make a soft dough. Tip out onto a lightly floured surface and lightly knead, fully incorporating any flour left in the bowl. Halve the mixture and flatten each piece to a rough oval, using your hands or a rolling pin, to a thickness of two £1 coins. Cut slashes through the centre of the ovals a couple of times with a sharp knife, being careful not to cut through an edge.

3 Heat a large non-stick pan, add a flatbread and cook for 1 min each side until firm and slightly puffed, then repeat with the other. Meanwhile, heat a large pan of water and poach the eggs to your liking.

4 Warm the beans and serve on top of each flatbread with a poached egg and some black pepper.

BENEFITS vegetarian • low fat • folate • iron • 3 of 5 a day
PER SERVING 550 kcals • fat 10g • saturates 3g •carbs 77g • sugars 28g • fibre 19g • protein 28g • salt 0.5g

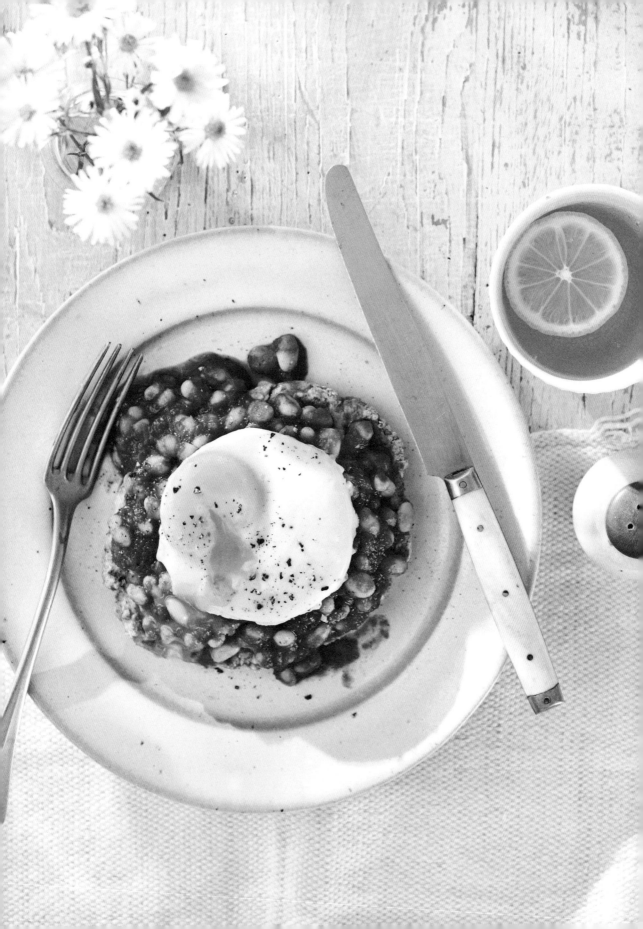

Banana Pancakes

Gluten-free banana pancakes you can whip up in just 10 minutes! Scatter with pecans and raspberries to enjoy a low-calorie yet indulgent breakfast.

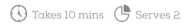 Takes 10 mins   Serves 2

- 1 large banana
- 2 medium eggs, beaten
- pinch of baking powder (gluten-free if coeliac)
- splash of vanilla extract
- 1 tsp rapeseed oil
- 25g/1oz pecans, roughly chopped
- 125g/4½oz raspberries

1 In a bowl, mash the banana with a fork until it resembles a thick purée. Stir in the eggs, baking powder and vanilla.

2 Heat a large non-stick frying pan or pancake pan over a medium heat and brush with half the oil. Using half the batter, spoon 2 pancakes into the pan, cook for 1-2 mins each side, then tip onto a plate. Repeat the process with the remaining oil and batter. Top the pancakes with the pecans and raspberries.

BENEFITS vegetarian • 1 of 5 a day • gluten free
PER SERVING 291 kcals • fat 10g • saturates 4g • carbs 40g • sugars 20g • fibre 5g • protein 7g • salt 0g

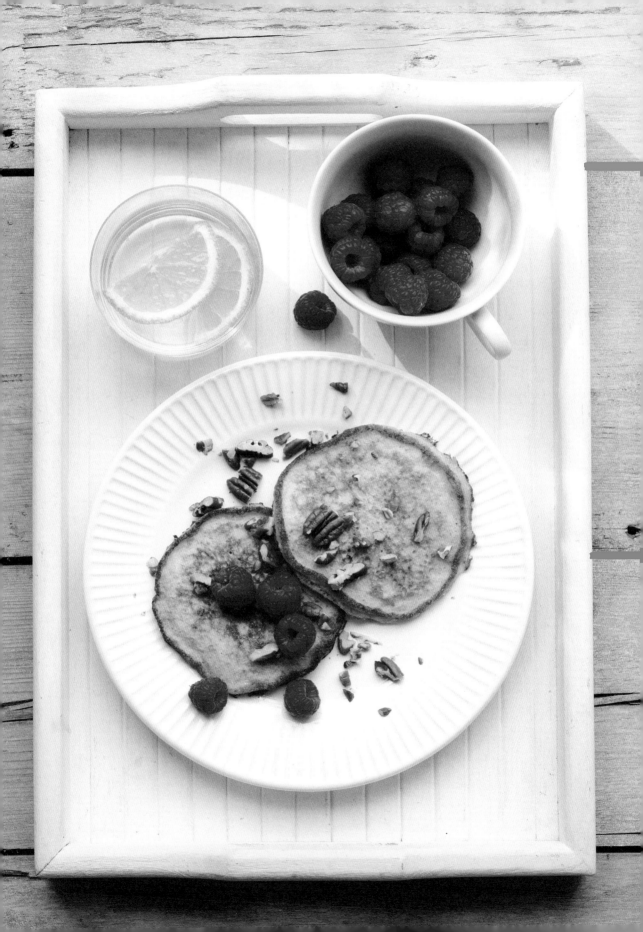

Pistachio Nut &
Spiced-apple Bircher

A balanced, filling breakfast bowl of oats and apple in yogurt spiced with cinnamon and nutmeg, topped with crunchy pomegranate seeds or juicy berries.

Takes 10 mins, plus overnight soaking Serves 2

FOR THE MUESLI BASE
- 50g/2oz porridge oats
- 50ml/2fl oz unsweetened apple juice
- large pinch of ground cinnamon
- large pinch of ground nutmeg
- 1 medium apple, cored and grated
- 2 tbsp live bio yogurt

FOR THE TOPPING
- 25g/1oz chopped pistachio nuts or almonds
- 3 tbsp pomegranate seeds or mixed berries

1 Mix all the muesli base ingredients, except the bio yogurt, with 150ml/¼ pint water and leave to soak for at least 20 minutes or overnight, if possible.
2 Once the oats have softened, stir through the yogurt, then divide the mixture between 2 bowls.
3 Sprinkle half of the topping over each bowl and serve.

TIP Cinnamon improves focus and attention, and regulates blood sugar levels.

BENEFITS *vegetarian •low cal • 1 of 5 a day*
PER SERVING 237 kcals • protein 8g • carbs 29g • fat 9g • saturates 2g • fibre 5g • sugars 14g • salt 0.1g

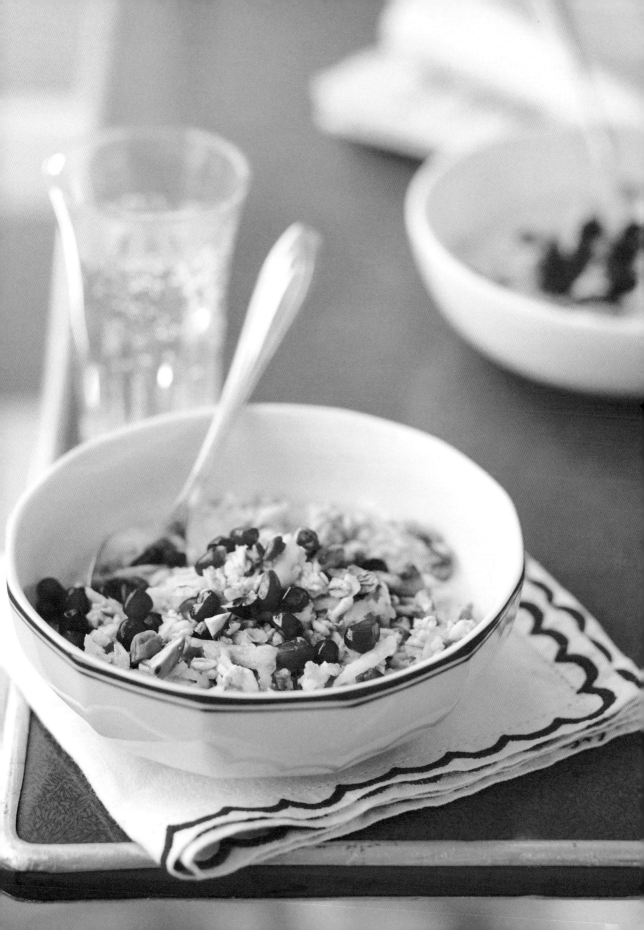

Herb Pancake Wraps with Goat's Cheese

Thin omelettes replace the usual flour tortillas here. They taste great warm or cold for a light lunch.

🕐 Takes 20 mins   🥧 Serves 2

- 1½ tsp rapeseed oil
- 2 spring onions, finely chopped
- 1 large courgette, coarsely grated and squeezed dry
- 2 large eggs
- 2 tbsp chopped basil
- 2 tsp thyme leaves
- 50g/2oz soft goat's cheese
- 2 medium tomatoes, chopped
- 6 Kalamata olives, rinsed and halved
- 2 handfuls baby kale or watercress
- radishes, to serve (optional)

1 Heat 1 tsp oil in a frying pan and add the spring onions and courgette. Cook, stirring frequently, to soften the courgette and drive off any excess moisture. Tip the veg into a bowl and wash the pan.

2 Beat an egg with 1 tbsp water, half the herbs and some black pepper. Heat the remaining rapeseed oil in the frying pan, pour in the egg mixture and swirl the pan to set it thinly on the base. Cook for a couple of mins, tip onto a plate and repeat with the other egg, 1 tbsp water and the remaining herbs.

3 Spread the goat's cheese down the centre of each pancake and top with the courgette mix, scatter over the tomatoes, olives and baby kale, then roll up and cut in half. Alternatively, spread the goat's cheese over the pancakes, top with the filling and serve open. Eat with some radishes on the side, if you like.

BENEFITS vegetarian • low cal • folate • vit c • 2 of 5 a day • gluten free
PER SERVING 254 kcals • fat 17g • saturates 7g • carbs 9g • sugars 5g • fibre 3g • protein 16g • salt 0.8g

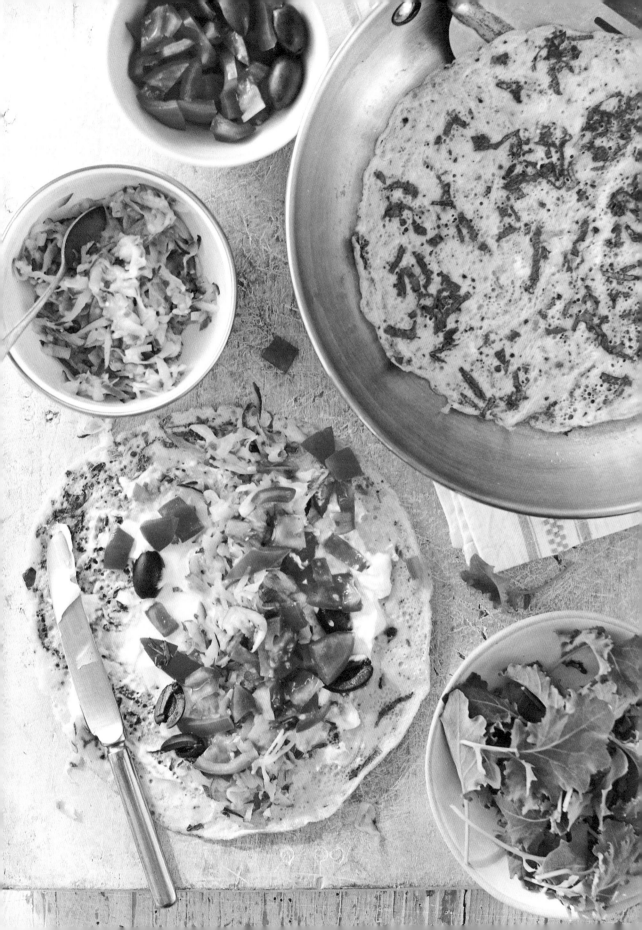

Summer Pistou

This is a cross between a soup and a stew, packed with veg and flavoured with aromatic basil. There will be enough for 2 days – simply keep in the fridge.

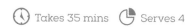 Takes 35 mins   Serves 4

- 1 tbsp rapeseed oil
- 2 leeks, finely sliced
- 1 large courgette, diced
- 1 litre/1¾ pints boiling vegetable stock (made with reduced-salt bouillon)
- 400g can cannellini or haricot beans, drained
- 200g/7oz green beans, chopped
- 3 tomatoes, chopped
- 3 garlic cloves, finely chopped
- small pack basil
- 40g/1½oz freshly grated Parmesan

1 Heat the oil in a large pan and fry the leeks and courgette for 5 mins to soften. Pour in the stock, add three-quarters of the cannellini beans with the green beans, half the tomatoes, and simmer for 5-8 mins until the vegetables are tender.

2 Meanwhile, blitz the remaining beans and tomatoes, the garlic and basil in a food processor (or in a bowl with a stick blender) until smooth, then stir in the Parmesan. Stir the sauce into the soup, cook for 1 min, then ladle half into bowls or pour into a flask for a packed lunch. Chill the remainder. Will keep for a couple of days.

BENEFITS vegetarian • low fat • fibre • vit c • 3 of 5 a day
PER SERVING 209 kcals • fat 8g • saturates 3g •carbs 18g • sugars 6g • fibre 10g • protein 12g • salt 0.2g

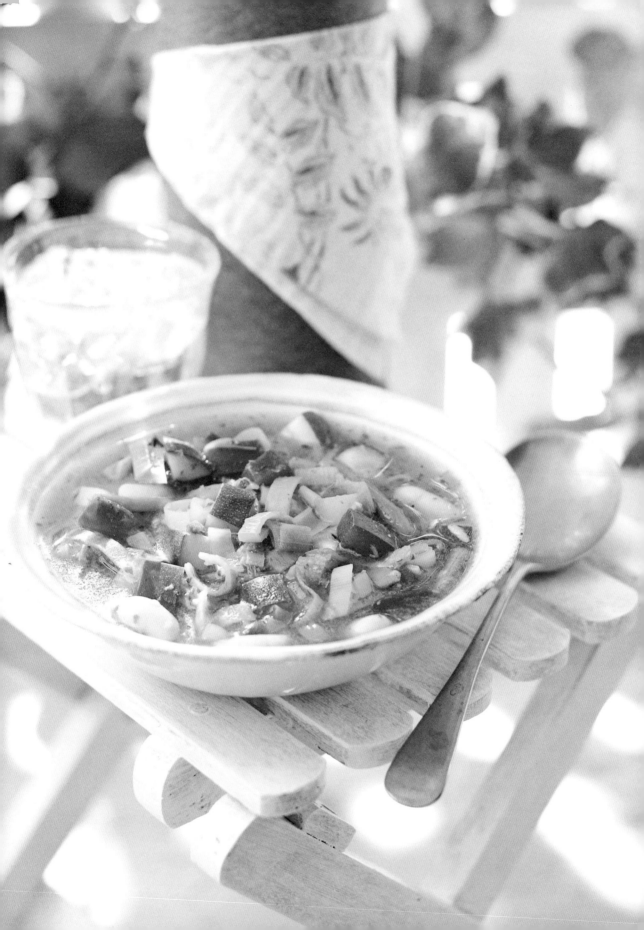

Peanut Houmous with Fruit & Veg Sticks

This houmous is perfect for spreading on crisp apple slices and celery or carrot sticks. Add extra liquid if you want a dipping consistency to serve with softer vegetables, such as chicory leaves, sugar snap peas and cucumber.

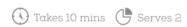 Takes 10 mins ⏲ Serves 2

- 380g carton chickpeas
- zest and juice ½ lemon (use the other ½ to squeeze over the apple to stop it browning, if you like)
- 1 tbsp tahini
- ½-1 tsp smoked paprika
- 2 tbsp roasted unsalted peanuts
- 1 tsp rapeseed oil
- 2 crisp red apples, cored and cut into slices
- 2 carrots, cut into sticks
- 4 celery sticks, cut into batons lengthways

1. Drain the chickpeas, reserving the liquid. Tip three-quarters of the chickpeas into a food processor and add the lemon zest and juice, tahini, paprika, peanuts and oil with 3 tbsp chickpea liquid.
2. Blitz in a food processor until smooth, then stir in the reserved chickpeas. Serve with the fruit and veg sticks.

TIP Celery is rich in compounds called coumarins that help lower blood pressure and maintain the body's water balance.

BENEFITS 4 of 5 a day
PER SERVING 336 kcals • fat 16g • saturates 2g • carbs 35g • sugars 16g • fibre 13g • protein 15g • salt 0.8g

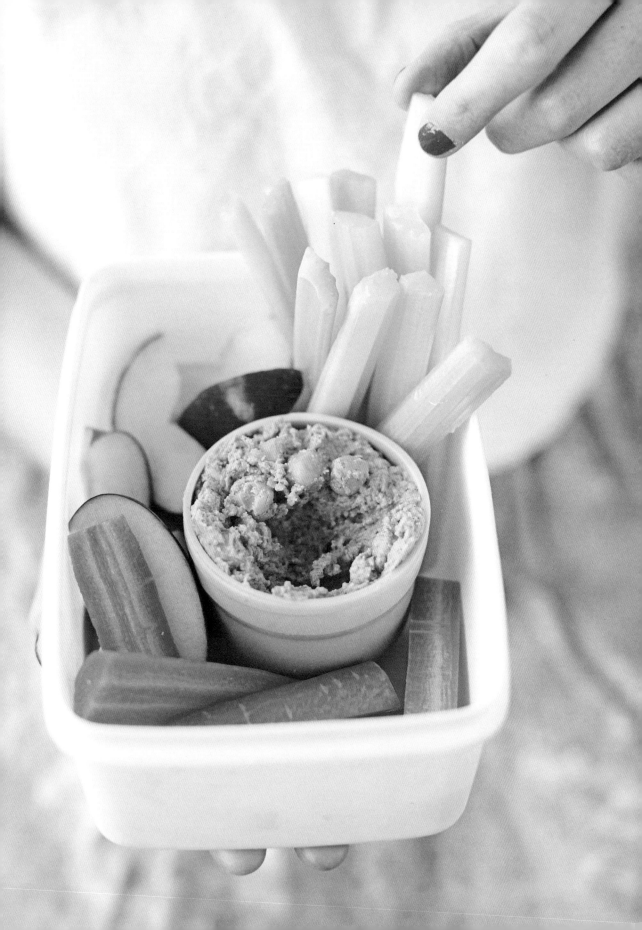

Barley Couscous & Prawn Tabbouleh

Barley couscous is a high fibre alternative to refined couscous. If you don't mind peeling them, look for Atlantic prawns in their shells, as they are not preserved in a salt glaze like their peeled equivalent.

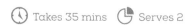 Takes 35 mins Serves 2

- 125g/4½oz barley couscous
- zest 1 lemon, juice of ½
- 1 tbsp extra virgin rapeseed or olive oil
- ½ small pack dill, finely chopped
- good handful mint leaves, chopped
- ½ cucumber, chopped
- 2 nectarines, chopped
- 125g/4½oz peeled prawns, if using prawns in their shells you need 250g/9oz

1 Tip the couscous into a bowl and pour over just enough boiling water to cover, following pack instructions. Leave for no more than 5 mins, drain thoroughly, then fluff up with a fork and tip into a bowl. Stir in the lemon zest and juice with the oil, dill and mint, then add the cucumber and nectarines.

2 Toss through the prawns and serve on plates or pack into lunch containers.

BENEFITS low fat • low cal • fibre • vit c • 2 of 5 a day
PER SERVING 393 kcals • fat 7g • saturates 1g •carbs 60g • sugars 13g • fibre 9g • protein 17g • salt 1.0g

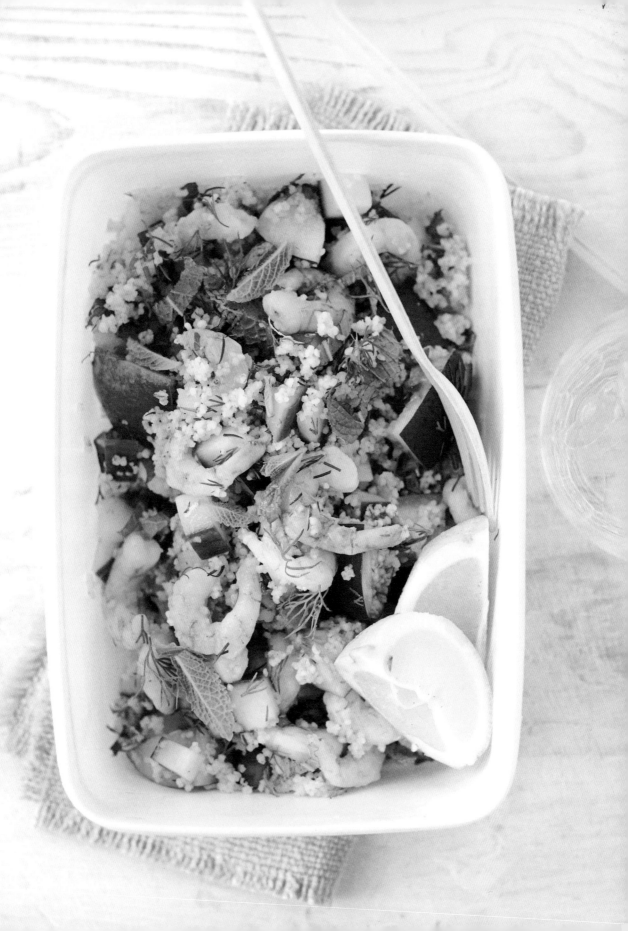

Asparagus & Lentil Salad with Crumbled Feta

Although packs of pre-cooked lentils are convenient, they often come with salt and extra flavourings, so it is well worth cooking your own.

🕐 Takes 30 mins   ◓ Serves 2

- 1 garlic clove
- 125g/4½oz Puy lentils
- 100g pack fine asparagus tips
- 3 spring onions, finely sliced
- 25g/1oz dried cranberries or raisins or freeze-dried raspberries
- 1 tbsp extra virgin rapeseed or olive oil, plus a little extra (optional)
- 2 tsp apple cider vinegar
- 140g/5oz cherry tomatoes, halved
- 50g/2oz feta

1 Finely grate the garlic and put in a bowl. Boil the lentils for 25 mins, and put the asparagus in a steamer over them for the last 5 mins until just tender.
2 Meanwhile, put the onions, cranberries, oil and vinegar in the bowl with the garlic and stir well. When the lentils are ready, drain and toss them into the dressing with the tomatoes. Tip into plastic containers (for a packed lunch), or onto plates, then top with the asparagus and crumble over the feta. Drizzle with a little extra oil, if you like.

TIP Spring onions and garlic are both sources of sulphur, which helps the liver to detoxify.

BENEFITS *vegetarian • folate • fibre • iron • 3 of 5 a day • gluten free*
PER SERVING *359 kcals • fat 12g • saturates 4g • carbs 35g • sugars 6g • fibre 11g • protein 22g • salt 1.0g*

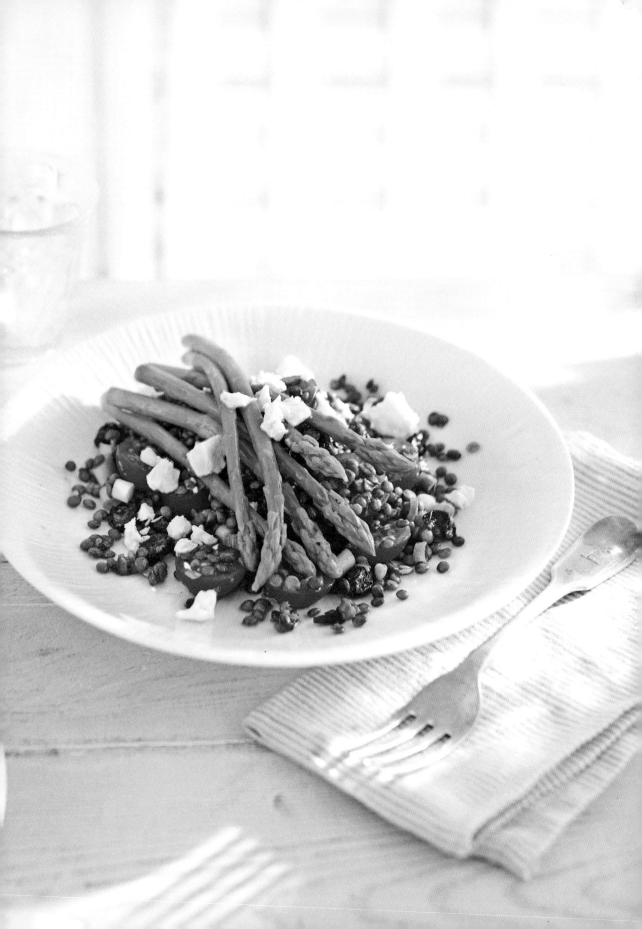

Super-green Soup with Yogurt & Pine nuts

This simple soup is a fresh new way to use a bag of mixed leaves, and freezes beautifully.

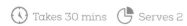 Takes 30 mins   Serves 2

- 2 tsp olive oil
- 1 onion, chopped
- 2 garlic cloves, crushed
- 1 potato (approx 250g/9oz), cut into small cubes
- 600ml/1 pint reduced-salt vegetable bouillion
- 120g bag mixed watercress, rocket and spinach salad
- 150g pot live bio yogurt
- 25g/1oz pine nuts, toasted chilli oil, to serve (optional)

1 Heat the oil in a medium saucepan over a low-medium heat. Add the onion and a pinch of salt, then cook slowly, stirring occasionally, for 10 mins until softened but not coloured. Add the garlic and cook for 1 min more.
2 Tip in the potato followed by the veg stock. Simmer for 10-12 mins until the potato is soft enough that a cutlery knife will slide in easily. Add the bag of salad and let it wilt for 1 min, then blitz the soup in a blender until it's completely smooth.
3 Serve with a dollop of yogurt, some toasted pine nuts and a drizzle of chilli oil, if you like.

TIP Spinach is rich in sun-protective carotenoids and antioxidants that protect against free radical damage.

BENEFITS *vegetarian • low fat • calcium • folate•fibre•vitc•1 of 5 a day*
PER SERVING *325 kcals • fat 13g • saturates 2g • carbs 36g • sugars 14g • fibre 7g • protein 12g • salt 1.0g*

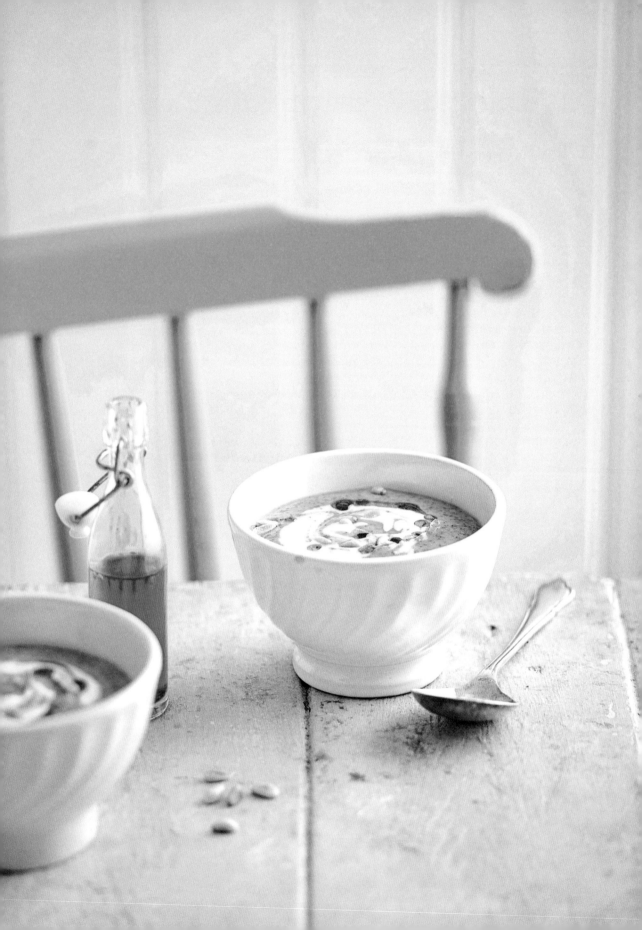

Baked Sweet Potatoes
with Lentils & Red Cabbage Slaw

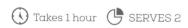

The spiced lentils will continue to thicken after they have been taken off the hob. If you're making this in advance, you'll need to add a little extra water when reheating.

🕐 Takes 1 hour   📖 SERVES 2

- 2 sweet potatoes (about 175g/6oz)
- 1 tbsp rapeseed oil
- 1 onion, finely sliced
- 2 garlic cloves, crushed
- thumb-sized piece ginger, peeled and finely grated
- 1 long green chilli, finely chopped (deseeded if you don't like it too hot)
- 2 tsp each ground cumin and ground coriander
- 85g/3oz split red lentils
- finely grated zest ½ lemon, plus 2 tbsp juice
- 2 tomatoes, chopped
- ½ small pack coriander, chopped, plus a few sprigs
- 4 tbsp live bio yogurt
- lemon wedges, for squeezing over (optional)

FOR THE RED CABBAGE SLAW
- 2 tbsp extra virgin olive oil
- 2 tsp lemon juice
- ¼ small red cabbage, cored and very finely sliced
- 1 carrot, peeled and grated
- 2 spring onions, finely sliced
- 25g/1oz sultanas
- 1 tbsp mixed seeds, such as sunflower, pumpkin, sesame and linseed

1 Heat oven to 220C/200C fan/gas 7. Put the washed and patted dry sweet potatoes on a baking tray and bake for 40 mins or until soft. Meanwhile, heat the oil in large non-stick saucepan over a medium-high heat. Fry the onion for 3-5 mins or until pale golden brown, stirring constantly, making sure it doesn't burn. Add the garlic, ginger, chilli and spices, and cook for a few secs, stirring constantly.

2 Add the lentils to the pan, pour over 400ml/14fl oz water, stir well and bring to the boil. Skim off any foam that rises to the surface with a spoon. Add ½ tsp flaked sea salt, the lemon zest and 1 tbsp of the lemon juice, stir well and reduce the heat to low.

3 Cover the pan loosely with a lid and leave to simmer gently for 20 mins or until the lentils are tender, stirring occasionally. Add the tomatoes, coriander and remaining 1 tbsp lemon juice, and cook for a further 5 mins, stirring. If the lentils thicken too much, add a splash of water. Season to taste.

4 To make the red cabbage slaw, whisk the oil and lemon juice together in a large bowl and season with lots of ground black pepper. Add the cabbage, carrot, spring onions, sultanas and seeds, then toss together well.

5 Put the potatoes on 2 plates, split them and fill with the lentils. Spoon over the yogurt, garnish with coriander and serve with the coleslaw and lemon wedges for squeezing over, if you like.

TIP Pumpkin seeds help to maintain healthy blood vessels and top up your calcium, magnesium and zinc intake.

BENEFITS vegetarian • calcium • folate • fibre • vit c • iron • 5 of 5 a day • gluten free
PER SERVING 752 kcals • fat 24g • saturates 4g • carbs 100g • sugars 53g • fibre 17g • protein 23g • salt 1.8g

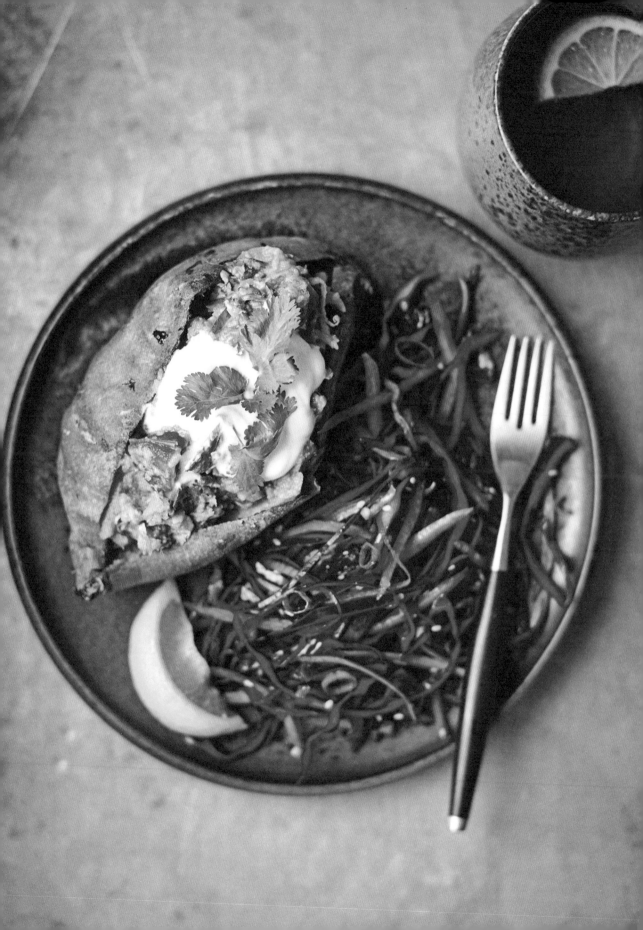

Crusted Polenta Tart
with Pesto, Courgette & Gruyère

A gluten-free polenta base makes this cheesy tart much lower in fat than traditional pastry - delicious served hot or cold for lunch the next day.

 Takes 1 hour 20 mins   Serves 4

FOR THE POLENTA CRUST

- 500ml/18 floz vegetable stock
- 140g/5oz fine polenta
- 50g/2oz Gruyère, finely grated
- 1 medium egg, lightly beaten
- 1 tbsp olive oil, for greasing

FOR THE TOPPING

- 3 tbsp pesto (see Pesto-crusted cod with Puy lentils page 150 for a homemade recipe)
- 3 small courgettes, thinly sliced
- 4 garlic cloves, finely sliced
- ½ small pack basil, leaves only
- 25g/1oz Gruyère, finely grated

1 First, make the polenta crust. Bring the vegetable stock to a simmer in a medium saucepan and, working quickly, pour the polenta into the pan. Keep your pan over a low heat and, using a wooden spoon, stir constantly, beating any lumps that form. Continue stirring for 5-6 mins until the polenta is very thick.

2 Remove the pan from the heat, add the Gruyère and stir until the cheese has melted. Finally, stir through the beaten egg, season generously, and allow to cool slightly.

3 Lightly brush a baking sheet with oil. Tip the polenta into the centre and, using a spatula or oiled fingers, gently spread the polenta into a rectangle shape roughly the size of an A4 sheet of paper.

4 Heat oven to 200C/180C fan/gas 6. Smother a thin layer of pesto over the polenta, leaving a 1-1.5cm/½in border around the edge of the tart. Top the pesto with slices of courgette, intermittently adding the sliced garlic and most of the basil. Season with ground black pepper and a good sprinkling of Gruyère.

5 Cook on the middle shelf of the oven for 45 mins. Reduce the temperature to 180C/160C fan/gas 4 for a further 15 mins. Remove and allow to cool for 5-10 mins, scatter over the remaining basil and serve.

BENEFITS vegetarian • low cal • 1 of 5 a day • gluten free
PER SERVING 322 kcals • fat 16g • saturates 6g • carbs 30g • sugars 3g • fibre 3g • protein 12g • salt 1.1g

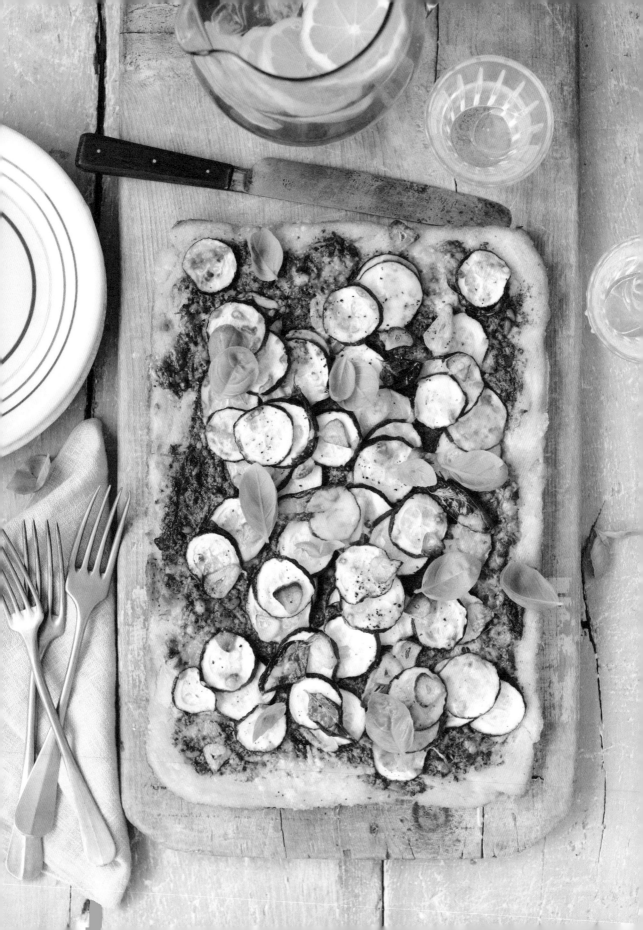

Niçoise Chicken Salad

We've given the usual tuna Niçoise a twist by using chicken, a lean meat that makes a filling substitute in this 3 of your 5 a day salad.

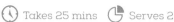 Takes 25 mins Serves 2

FOR THE DRESSING
- 2 tbsp rapeseed oil
- juice 1 lemon
- 1 tsp balsamic vinegar
- 1 garlic clove, grated
- ⅓ small pack basil, leaves chopped
- 3 pitted kalamata olives, rinsed and chopped

FOR THE SALAD
- 2 skinless chicken breasts
- 1 tsp rapeseed oil
- 250g/9oz new potatoes, thickly sliced
- 200g/7oz fine green beans
- ½ red onion, very finely chopped
- 14 cherry tomatoes, halved
- 6 romaine lettuce leaves, torn into bite-sized pieces
- 6 pitted Kalamata olives, rinsed and halved

1 Mix the dressing ingredients together in a small bowl with 1 tbsp water. Add 1 tbsp of the dressing to the chicken breasts and toss well to coat. Heat the oil in a small non-stick frying pan with a lid and cook the chicken for about 12 mins, covered, turning over halfway until cooked all the way through.
2 Meanwhile, boil the potatoes for 7 mins, add the green beans and boil for 5 mins more or until both are just tender, then drain.
3 Put the chicken on a plate to rest while you toss the beans, potatoes and remaining salad ingredients together in a large bowl with half the dressing. Slice the chicken, arrange on the salad, then add any juices to the remaining dressing and spoon on top.

BENEFITS low cal • folate • fibre • vit c • iron • 3 of 5 a day • gluten free
PER SERVING 471 kcals • fat 17g • saturates 2g • carbs 31g • sugars 11g • fibre 12g • protein 43g • salt 0.7 g

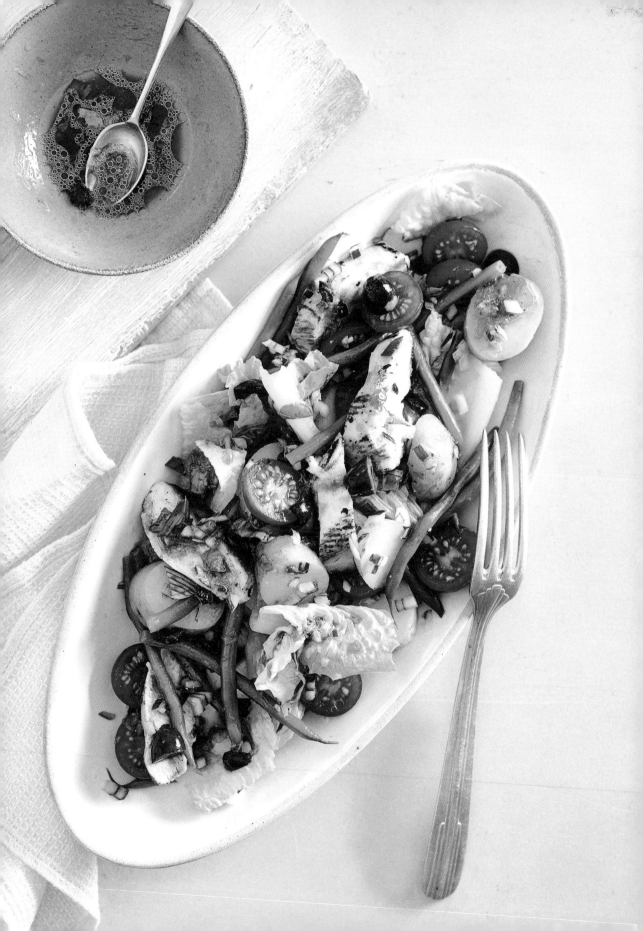

Chicken Spiralized Salad

Use a spiralizer or julienne peeler to create thin ribbons of cucumber and carrot for this fresh tasting salad. It's perfect for a take-to-work lunch.

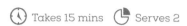 Takes 15 mins Serves 2

- ½ cucumber, spiralized or sliced into ribbons
- 2 carrots, spiralized or sliced into ribbons
- 100g bag crisp salad leaves (a mix of radicchio, frisée and round lettuce)
- 4 spring onions, finely sliced
- 200g cooked leftover roast chicken
- 2 tsp sesame seeds

FOR THE DRESSING
- 2 tbsp sesame oil
- 1½ tbsp cider apple vinegar
- 1½ tbsp wheat-free tamari
- ½ tbsp freshly grated ginger
- 1 tsp maple syrup

1 Layer all the salad ingredients into 2 plastic containers if you're packing to take to work, or put them in a large bowl.
2 Make the dressing by combining all the ingredients in a jar with a lid, add some seasoning and shake well. Put the dressing in 2 small pots to pack into your lunchboxes, or toss through the salad if eating straight away.

BENEFITS low fat • low cal • folate • 3 of 5 a day • gluten free
PER SERVING 284 kcals • fat 8g • saturates 1g • carbs 14g • sugars 12g • fibre 5g • protein 35g • salt 1.9g

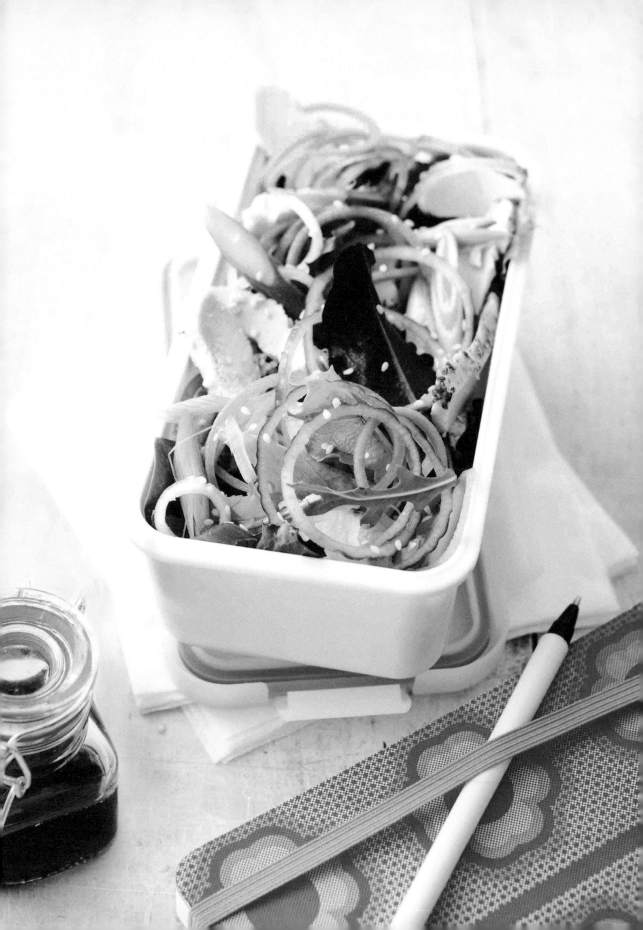

Wild Salmon Veggie Bowl

Succulent salmon flaked over a bed of healthy vegetables makes a delicious, protein-packed salad. Salmon is one of the oily varieties of fish that supplies beneficial omega-3 fats, which help maintain a sharp mind.

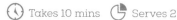 Takes 10 mins Serves 2

- 2 carrots
- 1 large courgette
- 2 cooked beetroots, diced
- 2 tbsp balsamic vinegar
- ⅓ small pack dill, chopped, plus some extra fronds (optional)
- 1 small red onion, finely chopped
- 280g poached or canned wild salmon
- 2 tbsp capers in vinegar, rinsed

1 Shred the carrots and courgette into strips with a julienne peeler or spiralizer, and pile onto 2 plates.
2 Stir the beetroot, balsamic vinegar, chopped dill and red onion together in a small bowl, then spoon on top of the veg. Flake over chunks of the salmon and scatter with the capers and extra dill, if you like.

BENEFITS low cal • calcium • folate • fibre • vit c • omega-3 •3 of 5 a day • gluten free
PER SERVING 395 kcals • fat 17g • saturates 4g • carbs 18g • sugars 16g • fibre 7g • protein 39g • salt 1.0g

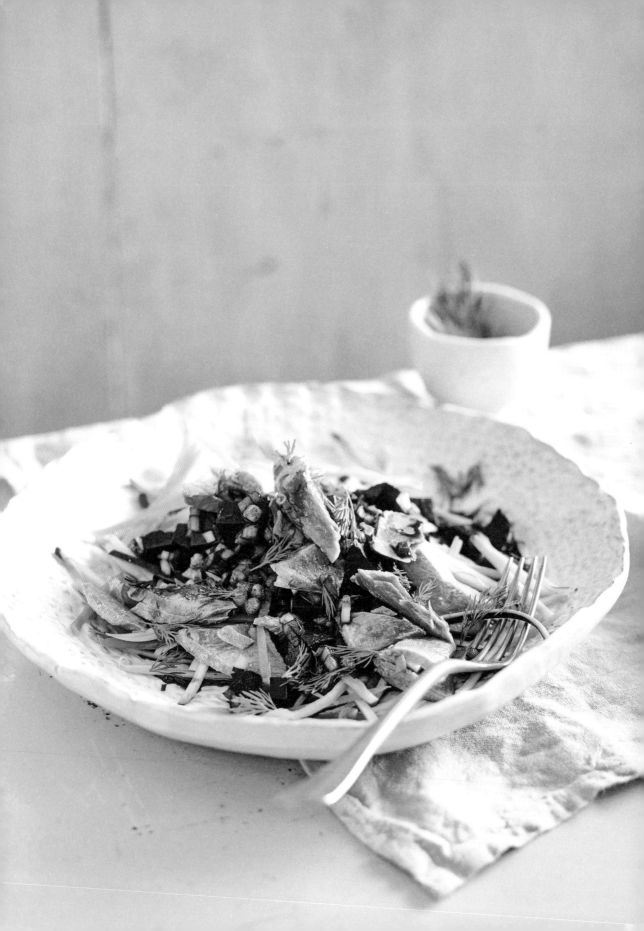

Asian Prawn & Cucumber Salad

This refreshing salad with its zing of lime and chilli heat makes a light and healthy lunch. If you haven't tried the protein-packed seed quinoa before, this is a great introduction – you can also use it instead of oats to make porridge.

 Takes 25 mins Serves 2

FOR THE SALAD
- 60g/2¼oz quinoa
- 150g/5½oz shelled North Atlantic prawns
- 1 small avocado, stoned and sliced
- ¼ cucumber, halved and sliced
- 5 Romaine lettuce leaves, torn into pieces
- 100g/4oz cherry tomatoes, halved

FOR THE DRESSING
- finely grated zest and juice 1 lime
- 1 red chilli, deseeded and finely chopped
- 2 spring onions, trimmed and finely chopped
- 1 tsp wheat-free tamari
- handful fresh coriander, chopped
- 1 tsp rapeseed oil
- ½ tsp maple syrup

1 Boil the quinoa in a small pan for 15 mins until the grains are tender and look like they have burst. Drain really well and tip into a bowl. Meanwhile, mix the lime zest and juice with 1 tbsp water and the chilli to make a dressing.

2 Stir half the dressing into the quinoa with the spring onion, tamari and half the chopped coriander and spoon onto 2 serving plates.

3 Stir the oil and maple syrup into the remaining dressing and toss in the prawns. Pile all the salad vegetables and the remaining coriander on top of the quinoa, spoon on the prawns with their dressing and serve.

BENEFITS low cal • iron • vit C • folate • fibre • 3 of 5 a day • gluten free,
PER SERVING 305 kcals • fat 14g • saturates 2g • carbs 22g • sugars 7g • fibre 7g • protein 19g • salt 1.5g

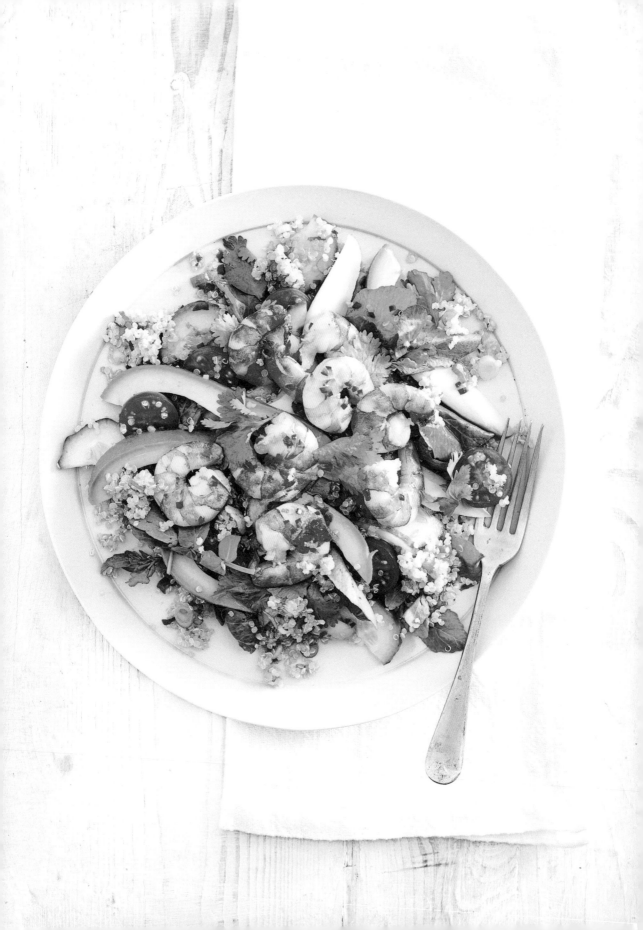

Chicken & Avocado Salad with Blueberry Dressing

Use leftover roast chicken or poach or pan-fry a chicken breast for this salad. Balsamic vinegar is worth having in your store cupboard; it really adds flavour to salad dressings.

🕐 Takes 20 mins   ◔ Serves 2

- 85g/3oz blueberries
- 1 tbsp rapeseed oil
- 2 tsp balsamic vinegar
- 125g/4½oz frozen baby broad beans or frozen soya beans
- 1 garlic clove, finely chopped
- 1 large cooked beetroot, finely chopped
- 1 avocado, halved, stoned, peeled and sliced
- 85g bag mixed baby leaf salad
- 175g/6oz cooked chicken, chopped

1 Mash half the blueberries with the oil, vinegar and some black pepper in a large salad bowl.
2 Boil the broad beans for 5 mins until just tender. Drain, leaving them unskinned.
3 Stir the garlic into the dressing, then pile in the warm beans and remaining blueberries with the beetroot, avocado, salad and chicken. Toss to mix, but don't go overboard or the juice from the beetroot will turn everything pink. Pile onto plates or into shallow bowls to serve.

BENEFITS low cal • fibre • 3 of 5 a day • gluten free
PER SERVING 402 kcals • fat 19g • saturates 3g • carbs 18g • sugars 10g • fibre 10g • protein 34g • salt 0.3g

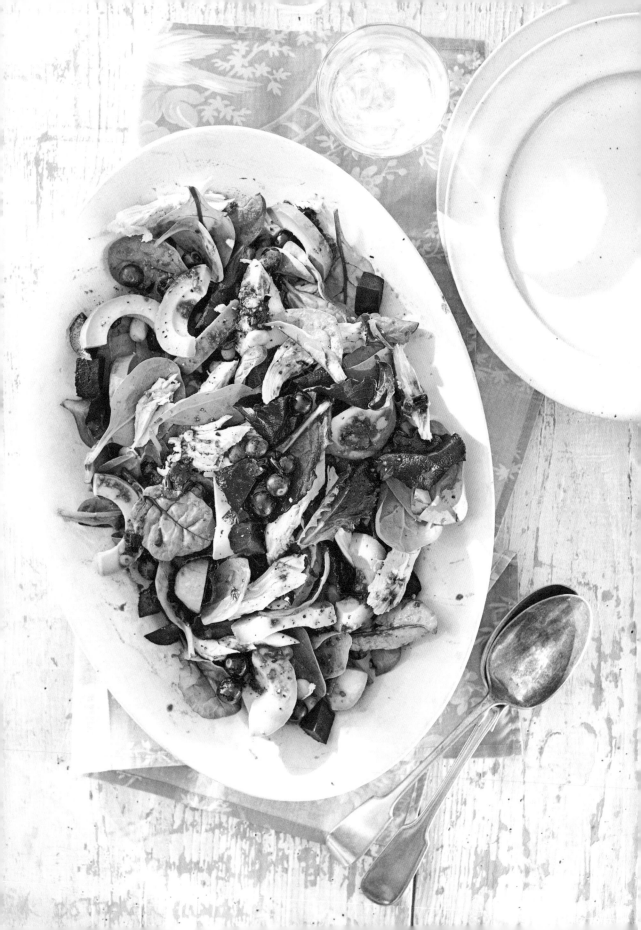

Lemon Pollock with Sweet Potato Chips

Frozen pollock fillets are really good value and are usually just labelled 'white fish fillets' in supermarkets. Served with sweet potato chips and a veg crush, this provides 3 of your 5 a day.

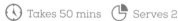 Takes 50 mins Serves 2

FOR THE CHIPS
- 1 garlic clove
- 2 sweet potatoes, scrubbed and cut into chips
- 2 tsp olive oil
- ½ tsp smoked paprika

FOR THE FISH & DRESSING
- 2 pollock fillets (about 100g/4oz each)
- 2 tbsp olive oil
- zest ½ lemon
- 1½ tsp capers, rinsed and chopped
- 1 tbsp chopped dill

FOR THE BROCCOLI MASH
- 1 leek, chopped
- 4 broccoli spears (about 200g/7oz)
- 85g/3oz frozen peas
- handful mint

1 Heat oven to 200C/180C fan/gas 6. Finely chop the garlic, put half in a bowl for the dressing and set the rest aside for the chips. Toss the sweet potatoes with the oil and spread out on a large baking sheet. Bake for 25 mins, turning halfway through.

2 Put the fish on a sheet of baking parchment on a baking sheet, brush with a little oil, then grate over the lemon zest and season with black pepper. Set aside.

3 Boil the leek for 5 mins, then add the broccoli and cook for 5 mins more. Tip in the peas for a further 2 mins. Drain, return them to the pan and blitz with a stick blender to make a thick purée. Add the mint, then blitz again.

4 Meanwhile, toss the reserved garlic and paprika with the chips and return to the oven with the fish for 10 mins. Add the olive oil to the garlic reserved for the dressing, with the capers and dill and 1 tbsp water. Serve everything together with the caper dressing spooned over the fish.

BENEFITS 3 of 5 a day • gluten free • fibre • vit c • folate
PER SERVING 531 kcals • fat 18g • saturates 3g • carbs 55g • sugars 28g • fibre 16g • protein 30g • salt 0.6g

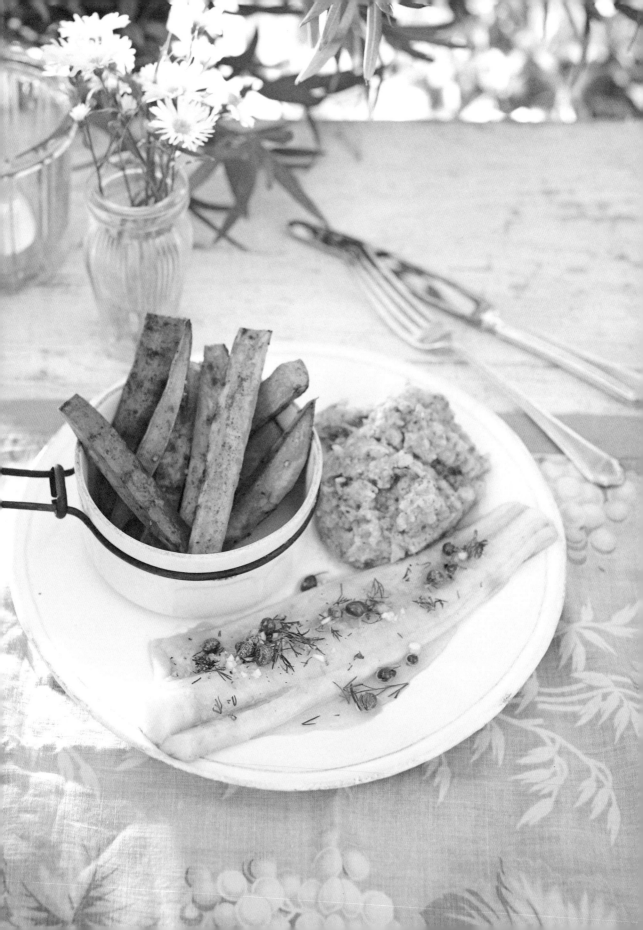

Salmon with Corn & Pepper Salsa Salad

Salmon coated in a spicy Mexican-style rub and served with a chunky salsa for a skin-boosting supper with 3 of your 5 a day.

 Takes 25 mins   Serves 2

FOR THE SPICY SALMON
- 1 garlic clove
- ½ tsp mild chilli powder
- ½ tsp ground coriander
- ¼ tsp ground cumin
- 1 lime, grated zest and juice, plus wedges to serve (optional)
- 2 tsp rapeseed oil
- 2 skinless salmon fillets, preferably wild

FOR THE SALSA SALAD
- 1 corn on the cob
- 1 red onion, finely chopped
- 1 avocado, halved, stoned, peeled and finely chopped
- 1 red pepper, deseeded and finely chopped
- 1 red chilli, halved, deseeded and chopped
- ½ pack coriander, finely chopped

1 Finely grate the garlic into a bowl for the spice rub. Boil the corn for the salsa salad for 6-8 mins until tender, then drain and cut off the kernels with a sharp knife.
2 Stir the spices, 1 tbsp lime juice and the oil into the garlic to make a spice rub, then use to coat the salmon.
3 Mix the remaining lime zest and juice into the corn and stir in all the remaining ingredients. Heat a frying pan and cook the salmon for 2 mins each side so that it is still a little pink in the centre. Serve with the salsa salad with extra lime wedges, if you like, for squeezing over.

BENEFITS omega-3 • folate • fibre • vit c • 3 of 5 a day • gluten free
PER SERVING 530 kcals • fat 32g • saturates 5g • carbs 27g • sugars 12g • fibre 9g • protein 29g • salt 0.2g

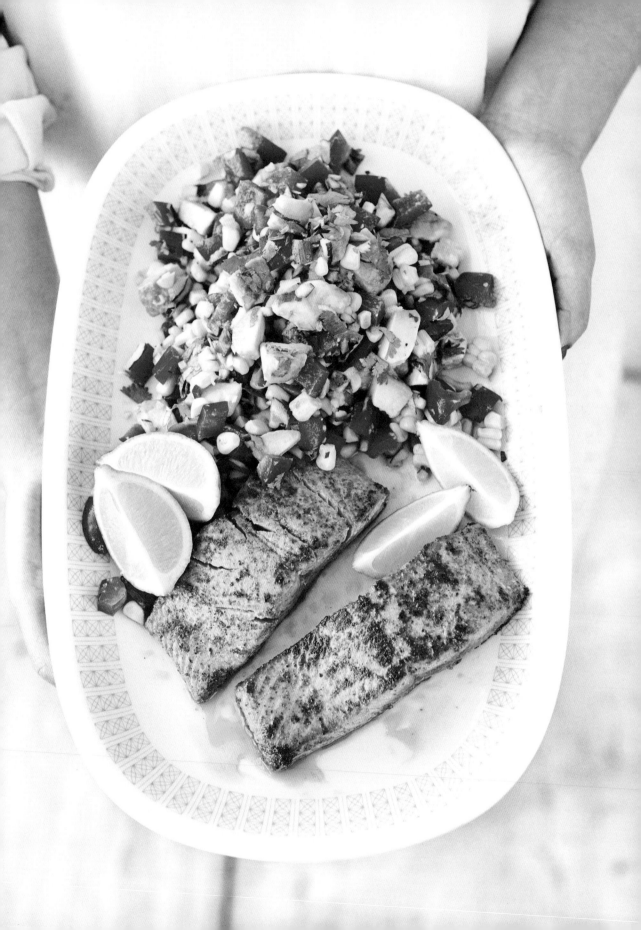

Herby Lamb Fillet with Caponata

A delicious Sunday roast can be healthy, as this low-calorie recipe proves. It contains an amazing 5 of your 5 a day, and provides fibre, vitamins and minerals.

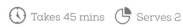 Takes 45 mins　　Serves 2

- 3 garlic cloves

FOR THE CAPONATA
- 2 tsp rapeseed oil
- 1 red onion, cut into wedges
- 1 aubergine, sliced and quartered
- 500g carton passata
- 1 green pepper, quartered, deseeded and sliced
- 6 pitted Kalamata olives, halved and rinsed
- 2 tsp capers, rinsed
- 1 tsp chopped rosemary
- 1 tsp balsamic vinegar

FOR THE LAMB & POTATOES
- 4 baby new potatoes, halved
- 1 tsp chopped rosemary
- 1 tsp rapeseed oil
- 250g/9oz lean lamb loin fillet, all visible fat removed
- 240g bag baby spinach
- finely chopped parsley (optional)

1 Slice 2 garlic cloves for the caponata, finely grate the other for the lamb and set aside. Heat the oil for the caponata in a wide pan, add the onion and fry for 5 mins to soften. Tip in the aubergine and cook, stirring, for 5 mins more. Add the passata and pepper with the olives, capers, rosemary and balsamic vinegar, then cover and cook for 15 mins, stirring frequently.

2 Meanwhile, heat oven to 190C/170C fan/gas 5. Boil the potatoes for 10 mins, then drain. Mix the grated garlic with the rosemary and some black pepper, then rub all over the lamb. Toss the potatoes in the oil with some more black pepper, place in a small roasting tin with the lamb and roast for 15-20 mins. Meanwhile, wilt the spinach in the microwave or in a pan, and squeeze to drain any excess liquid.

3 Stir the garlic into the caponata and serve with the lamb, either whole or sliced, rolled in parsley if you like, with the potatoes and spinach.

BENEFITS low fat • low cal • calcium • folate • fibre • vit c • iron • 5 of 5 a day • gluten free
PER SERVING 483 kcals • fat 17g • saturates 5g • carbs 40g • sugars 24g • fibre 17g • protein 34g • salt 1.4g

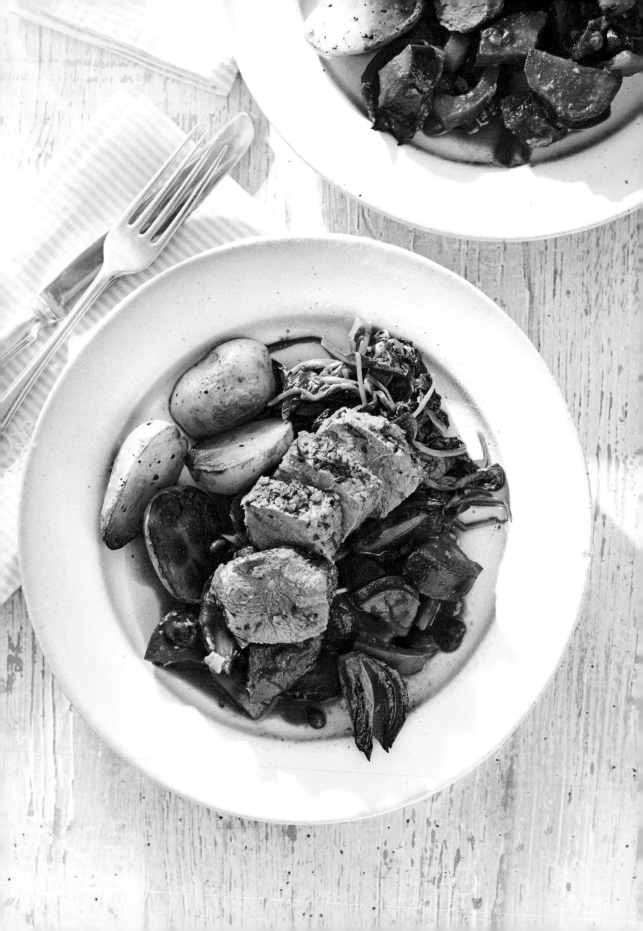

Spicy Vegetable Pilau with Cucumber Raita

Instead of the more traditional rice, this uses freekeh, a green wheat that has been roasted then cracked.

 Takes 40 mins   Serves 2

FOR THE PILAU
- 2 garlic cloves
- 1 tbsp rapeseed oil
- 1 large onion, quartered and sliced
- thumb-sized piece ginger, chopped
- 1 cinnamon stick
- ½ tsp cumin seeds
- seeds from 8 cardamom pods
- 1 tsp each ground turmeric and coriander
- 1 red chilli, halved, deseeded and sliced
- 1 large red pepper, deseeded and diced
- 50g/2oz freekeh
- 350ml/12fl oz vegetable bouillion (made with 2 tsp reduced-salt bouillon powder)
- 25g/1oz sultanas
- ½ pack coriander, chopped
- 40g/1½oz cashew nuts

FOR THE RAITA
- 1 garlic clove
- 150ml pot live bio yogurt
- ¼ cucumber, grated
- 2 tbsp chopped mint

1 Chop the garlic for the pilau and set aside. Finely grate the garlic for the raita and put in a bowl. Heat the oil for the pilau in a large open pan, and fry the onion and ginger for 5 mins until softened. Stir in the whole and ground spices, and cook for a few secs to release their aromas. Add the chilli, red pepper and freekeh, stir briefly, then tip in the stock and sultanas. Simmer for 15 mins until the freekeh is tender but still nutty, adding the chopped garlic for the final 2 mins. The stock should have reduced and absorbed into the freekeh now.
2 Meanwhile, finish the raita by stirring the yogurt, cucumber and mint into the grated garlic.
3 When the pilau is cooked, stir in the coriander and cashews, and serve with the raita.

TIP Rich in vitamin C, peppers help to maintain the skin's natural scaffolding system – collagen.

BENEFITS vegetarian • low cal • calcium • folate • fibre • vit c • iron • 3 of 5 a day
PER SERVING 471 kcals • fat 20g • saturates 4g • carbs 53g • sugars 27g • fibre 7g • protein 17g •
salt 0.2g

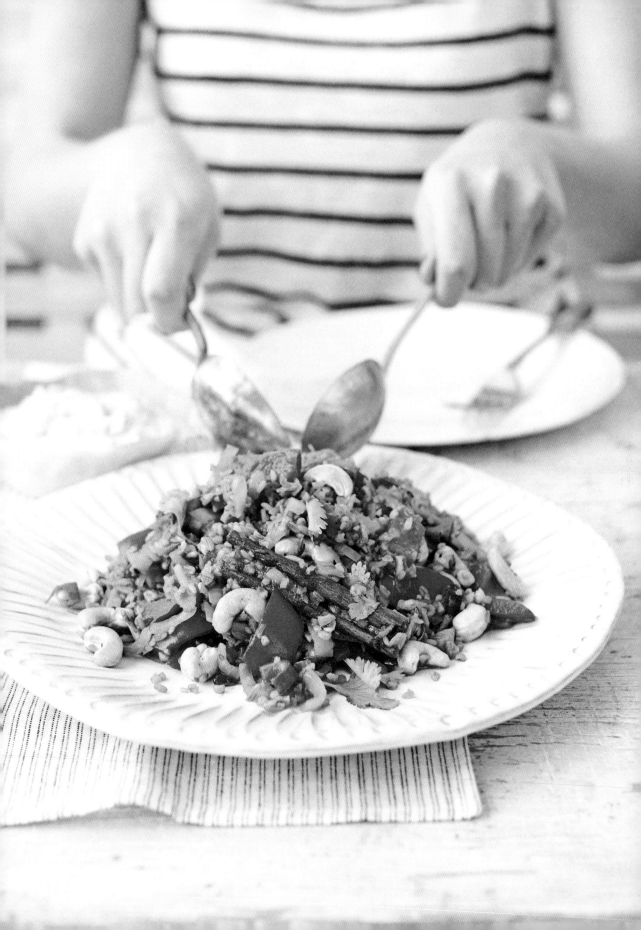

Veggie Meatballs with Tomato Courgetti

Instead of tossing into pasta, these veggie meatballs are accompanied by the lighter option of courgetti. Using ground almonds instead of breadcrumbs increases the protein and essential fats; it also means they're gluten-free.

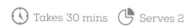 Takes 30 mins   Serves 2

- 3 garlic cloves

FOR THE VEGGIE MEATBALLS
- 2 tsp rapeseed oil, plus extra for greasing
- 1 small onion, very finely chopped
- 2 tsp balsamic vinegar
- 100g/4oz cooked red kidney beans (canned is fine)
- 1 tbsp beaten egg
- 1 tsp tomato purée
- 1 heaped tsp chilli powder
- ½ tsp ground coriander
- 15g/½oz ground almonds
- 40g/1½oz cooked sweetcorn
- 2 tsp chopped thyme leaves

FOR THE TOMATO COURGETTI
- 2 large or 3 normal tomatoes, chopped
- 1 tsp tomato purée
- 1 tsp balsamic vinegar
- 2 courgettes cut into 'noodles' with a spiralizer, julienne peeler or by hand

1 Finely chop the garlic. Heat the oil in a large pan and fry the onion, stirring frequently, for 8 mins. Stir in the balsamic vinegar and cook for 2 mins more. Meanwhile, put the beans in a bowl with the egg, tomato purée and spices, and mash until smooth. Stir in the almonds and sweetcorn with the thyme, a third of the chopped garlic and the balsamic onions. Mix well and shape into about 8 balls the size of a walnut, and place on a baking tray lined with oiled baking parchment.

2 Heat oven to 220C/200C fan/gas 7 and bake the veggie meatballs for 15 mins until firm. Meanwhile, put the tomatoes, tomato purée and balsamic vinegar in a pan and cook with 2-3 tbsp water until pulpy, then stir in the remaining garlic and courgetti. Turn off the heat as you want to warm the noodles rather than cook them. Serve with the veggie meatballs.

TIP Almonds are rich in brain-friendly omega-3 fatty acids and protective vitamin E.

BENEFITS vegetarian • low fat • low cal • folate • fibre • vit c • 3 of 5 a day • gluten free
PER SERVING 258 kcals • fat 11g • saturates 1g • carbs 24g • sugars 12g • fibre 9g • protein 12g • salt 0.7g

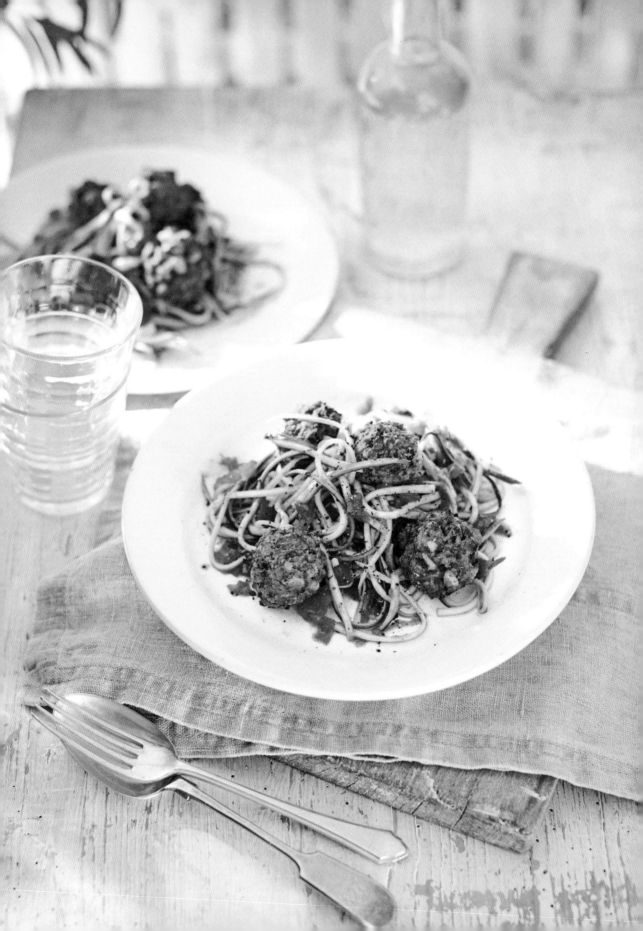

Roast Chicken with Sweet Potato Gremolata Salad

Roast a whole chicken for this recipe and use the rest later in the week– or you could use 140g/5oz pre-cooked chicken, or poach a large breast instead.

🕐 Takes 1 hours 25 mins   🥧 Serves 2

- 1 lemon
- 1.5kg/3lb 5oz whole chicken (free-range or organic), fat from inside the neck cavity removed
- 3 tbsp finely chopped parsley leaves (reserve the stalks)
- 2 sweet potatoes (175g/6oz each)
- 2 red onions, cut into wedges
- 1 tsp fennel seeds
- 7 whole garlic cloves
- 2 tsp extra virgin rapeseed or olive oil
- 125g bag baby spinach, washed
- 4 heaped tbsp pomegranate seeds

1 Heat oven to 200C/180C fan/gas 6. Grate the zest and squeeze the juice from the lemon into 2 bowls, then push the wedges inside the cavity of the chicken with the parsley stalks. Put the chicken in a roasting tin and roast for 30 mins.

2 Meanwhile, scrub the sweet potatoes (no need to peel) and cut into chunks. Put in another roasting tin with the onions, fennel, and 6 whole garlic cloves, then toss with the oil. When the chicken has had its 30 mins, put the potatoes in the oven and roast for 30-40 mins more.

3 Meanwhile, finely chop the remaining garlic clove for the gremolata, then mix with the lemon zest and parsley. Mix the lemon juice, oil and some black pepper in a bowl.

4 Remove the chicken and potatoes from the oven. Cover the chicken and leave to rest. Stir half the gremolata mix into the lemon juice and oil. Stir the spinach through the potato mix and return to the oven for 2 mins to wilt. Tip into the lemon dressing and toss well. Carve a chunk of breast meat from the chicken (you need about 140g), remove the skin, then cut into pieces. Toss into the salad with the pomegranate seeds, then serve scattered with the remaining gremolata.

TIP Pomegranate seeds are packed with protective polyphenols, which help to hydrate and regulate the skin's blood flow, promoting a rosy glow.

BENEFITS low fat • low cal • calcium • folate • fibre • vit c • iron • 3 of 5 a day • gluten free
PER SERVING 477 kcals • fat 8g • saturates 1g • carbs 65g • sugars 37g • fibre 14g • protein 29g •
salt 0.6g

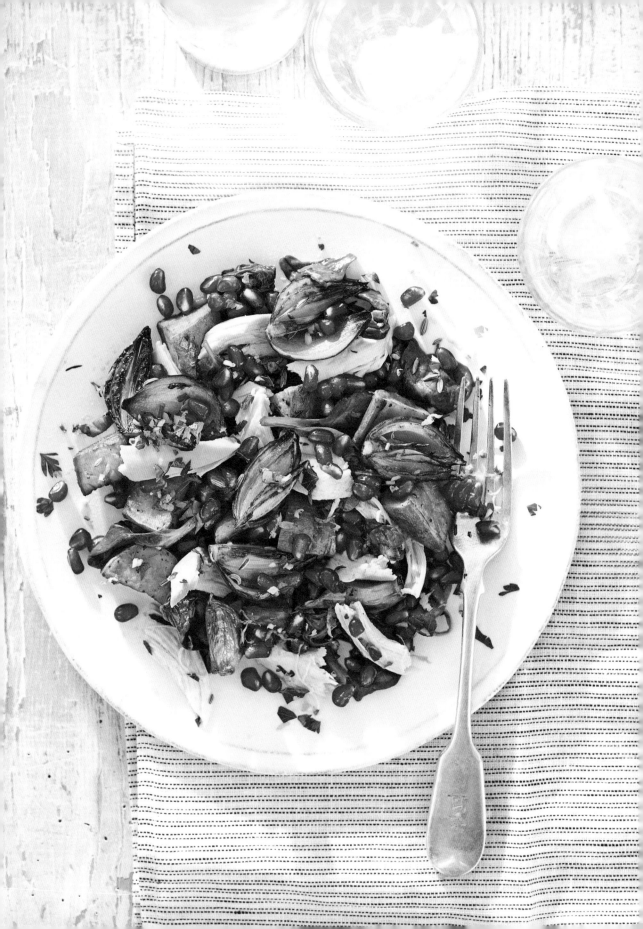

Wholewheat Pasta
with Broccoli & Almonds

Brown spaghetti keeps you fuller for longer, supplying slow release carbs - team it with healthy greens flavoured with garlic, chilli and lemon.

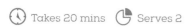 Takes 20 mins Serves 2

- 2 tbsp extra virgin rapeseed or olive oil
- 1 red chilli, deesed and sliced
- 3 garlic cloves, thinly sliced
- 250g/9oz wholewheat spaghetti
- 300g/11oz thin-stemmed broccoli, cut into pieces
- zest 1 lemon
- 25g/1oz flaked toasted almonds
- Parmesan shavings or vegetarian alternative, to serve

1 Bring a large pan of salted water to the boil. Meanwhile, heat the oil in a large frying pan. Add the chilli and garlic, and cook on a low heat until golden. Remove from the heat.

2 Add the pasta to the water and cook following pack instructions. In the final 4 mins of cooking, add the broccoli. Once cooked, drain and tip into the garlic pan. Add the lemon zest and almonds, and toss together well. Serve in bowls, topped with Parmesan shavings.

BENEFITS vegetarian • folate • fibre • vit c • 1 of 5 a day
PER SERVING 638 kcals • fat 23g • saturates 3g • carbs 82g • sugars 6g • fibre 16g • protein 26g • salt 0g

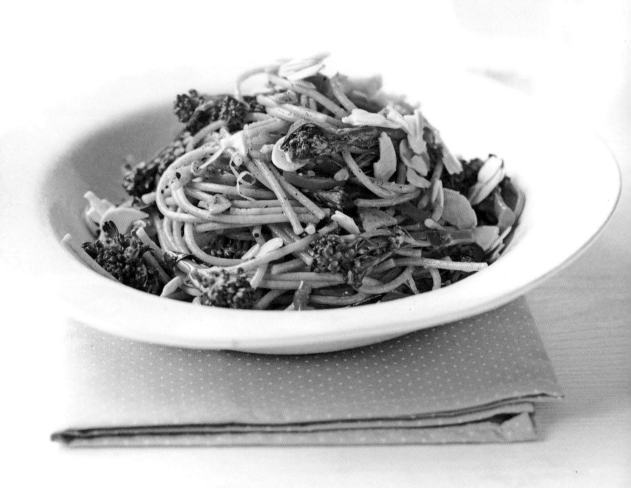

Quinoa Veggie Stir-fry

Tamari, a wheat-free alternative to soy sauce, is naturally salty. You might be surprised to see limes in here but, like lemons, they have an alkalising effect on the body when they're digested.

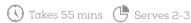 Takes 55 mins   Serves 2-3

- 100g/4oz quinoa
- 1 tbsp sesame oil
- 1 small red onion, thinly sliced
- 1 garlic clove, grated
- thumb-sized piece ginger, grated
- ½ tsp ground coriander
- 1 tbsp wheat-free tamari
- 1 red pepper, deseeded and sliced
- 100g/4oz green beans, tailed and cut in half
- 1 large courgette, sliced
- 2 tbsp sesame seeds
- small pack coriander, roughly chopped

FOR THE DRESSING
- zest and juice 2 limes
- pinch of pink Himalayan salt
- 2 tbsp sesame oil
- ½ garlic clove, crushed
- ½ tsp apple cider vinegar
- 1 tsp wheat-free tamari

1 Cook the quinoa following pack instructions and leave to cool.
2 In a large frying pan or wok, pour in the sesame oil and add the onion, garlic, ginger, ground coriander and tamari and fry on a medium-high heat for 2 mins until the moisture starts to evaporate, then add 3 tbsp water. Leave to fry for 1 min more, add the pepper and fry for another 2 mins.
3 Add 4 tbsp water, fry for another 2 mins, then add another 250ml/9fl oz water. After another 2 mins, add the green beans and another 125ml/4½fl oz water.
4 After another 2 mins, add the courgette, 125ml/4½fl oz water and leave to cook for 3 mins, then take off the heat.
5 Make the dressing by putting all the ingredients in a jug and whisking until smooth. Mix the quinoa into the veg, add the dressing and mix together with the sesame seeds. Stir through the coriander to serve.

BENEFITS vegetarian • low cal • folate • fibre • vit c • iron • 3 of 5 a day • gluten free
PER SERVING (2) 465 kcals • fat 25g • saturates 4g • carbs 40g • sugars 14g • fibre 7g • protein 16g • salt 1.8g

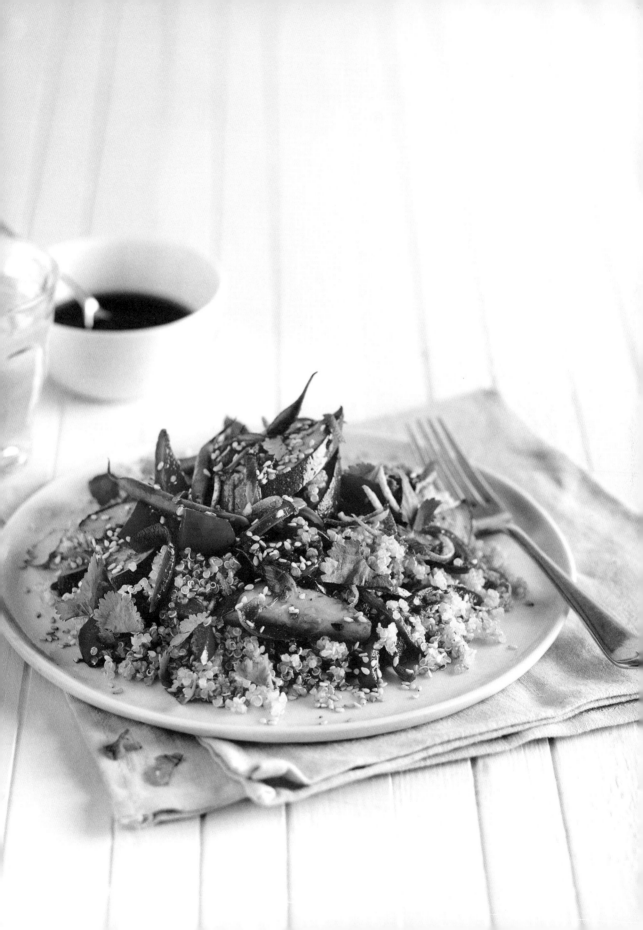

Steak, Roasted-pepper & Pearl-barley Salad

A vibrant salad with yellow and red peppers – bursting with skin-friendly vitamin C, anti-inflammatory onion, beef cooked to your liking and healthy grains.

🕐 Takes 40 minutes ◐ Serves 2

- 85g/3oz pearl barley, rinsed
- 1 red pepper, deseeded and cut into strips
- 1 yellow pepper, deseeded and cut into strips
- 1 red onion, cut into 8 wedges, leaving root intact
- 1 tbsp rapeseed or olive oil, plus a little extra
- 1 large lean beef steak, about 300g/11oz, trimmed of any excess fat
- ½ x 100g bag watercress, roughly chopped
- juice ½ lemon, plus wedges to garnish (optional)

1 Put the pearl barley in a large pan of water. Bring to the boil and cook vigorously for 25–30 mins or until tender. Drain thoroughly and transfer to a bowl. Set aside.

2 Meanwhile, heat oven to 200C/180C fan/gas 6. Put the peppers in a roasting tin with the onion wedges, toss in the oil and roast for about 20 mins until tender.

3 While the peppers are roasting, rub the steak with a little bit of extra oil and season. Cook in a non-stick frying pan for 3–4 mins each side, or to your liking. Leave to rest for a few mins.

4 Mix the cooked peppers and onions into the barley. Stir though the watercress, lemon juice and some seasoning, then transfer to a serving plate. Thinly slice the steaks, put on top of the salad and serve with lemon wedges to squeeze over, if you like.

TIP Watercress is a good source of vitamin K and calcium – both key for maintaining strong healthy bones.

BENEFITS low cal • folate • vit c • iron • 3 of 5 a day
PER SERVING 498 kcals • fat 17g • saturates 5g • carbs 48g • sugars 13g • fibre 6g • protein 38g • salt 0.2g

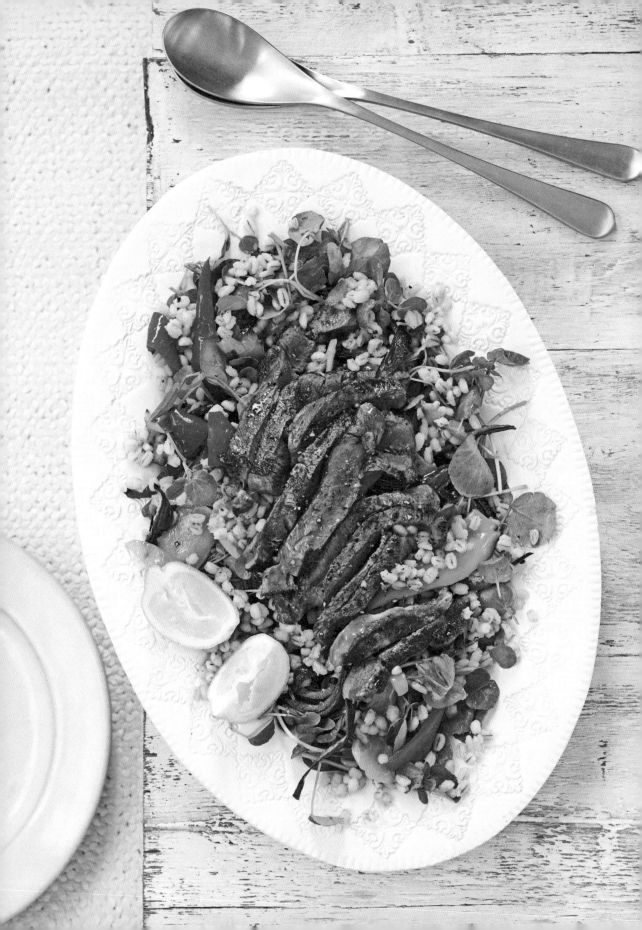

Creamy Chicken & Asparagus Braise

There is more to eating your greens than you might realise and they don't have to be leafy. Asparagus is richer in brain-friendly folate than broccoli, and supplies chromium, which helps to balance our blood sugar levels.

🕐 Takes 30-35 mins   ◖ Serves 2

- 1 tbsp rapeseed oil
- 2 skinless chicken breasts
- 10 medium asparagus spears, each cut into 3
- 1 large or 2 small leeks, well washed and thickly sliced
- 3 celery sticks, sliced
- 200ml/7fl oz reduced-salt vegetable bouillon
- 140g/5oz frozen peas
- 1 egg yolk
- 4 tbsp live bio yogurt
- 1 garlic clove, finely grated
- ⅓ small pack fresh tarragon, chopped
- new potatoes, to serve (optional)

1 Heat the oil in a large non-stick frying pan and fry the chicken for 5 mins, turning to brown both sides.

2 Add the asparagus (reserve the tips), leeks and celery, pour in the bouillon and simmer for 10 mins. Add the asparagus tips and peas, and cook for 5 mins more.

3 Meanwhile, stir the egg yolk with the yogurt and garlic. Stir the yogurt mixture into the vegetables and add the tarragon. Divide between 2 warm plates, then place the chicken on top of the vegetables. Serve with new potatoes, if you like.

TIP Peas are a useful source of iron and fibre, including soluble fibre, which helps regulate cholesterol levels.

BENEFITS *low fat • low cal • calcium • folate • fibre • vit c • iron • 3 of 5 a day*
PER SERVING *480 kcals • fat 15g • saturates 4g • carbs 25g • sugars 18g • fibre 15g • protein 53g • salt 0.5g*

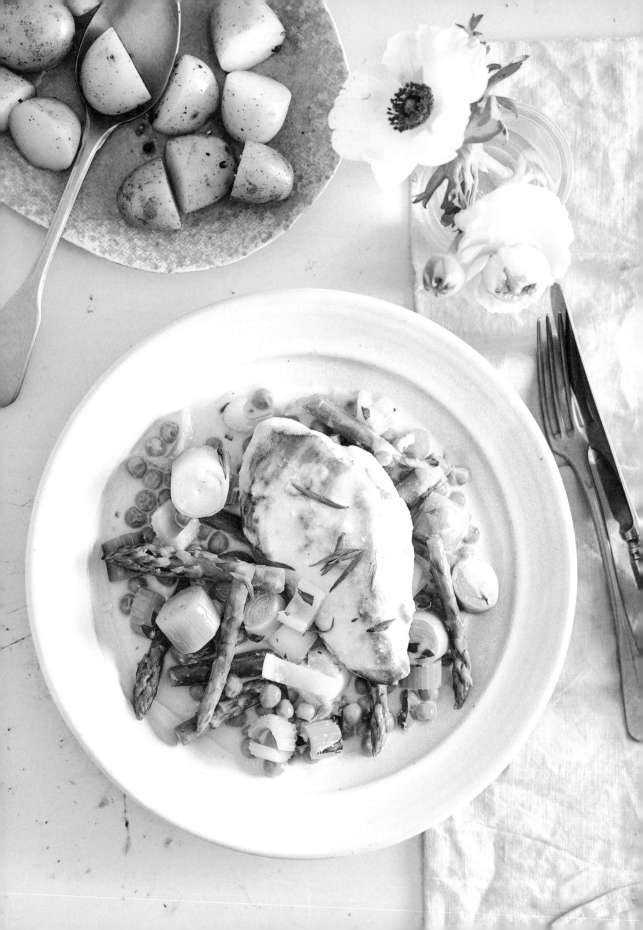

Indian Spiced Chicken with Squash & Beans

Good digestion is one of the cornerstones of our wellbeing and this recipe with butternut squash is a source of cleansing fibre and easily absorbed carotenoids that may protect gains some cancers and eye disease.

Takes 55 mins, plus marinating   Serves 2

- 150ml/¼ pint bio live yogurt
- 1 tbsp finely grated ginger
- ½ tsp ground turmeric
- 1 tsp ground cumin
- 4 skinless chicken thigh fillets (about 250g/9oz), cut into big chunks
- 200g/7oz butternut squash, cut into bite-sized chunks
- 1 tbsp coconut or rapeseed oil
- 2 red onions, halved and thickly sliced
- 1 garlic clove
- 4 sprigs mint, leaves picked
- 25g/1oz coriander, chopped
- 300g can red kidney beans, drained and rinsed
- grated zest and juice ½ lime
- 1 head of chicory, thickly sliced

1 Put 2 tbsp of the yogurt in a bowl with the spices, chicken and a really good grinding of black pepper, and set aside for 30 mins, or longer if you have time, to marinate.

2 Heat oven to 200C/180C fan/gas 6. Arrange the squash on a large baking tray, crumble over the coconut oil (as it will be solid at this stage) and roast for 20 mins. Add the onions and chicken, spaced apart, and roast for 20 mins more until everything is cooked.

3 Meanwhile, put the rest of the yogurt in a bowl with the garlic, mint and two-thirds of the coriander, and blitz with a stick blender until smooth. Tip the beans and remaining coriander into a bowl, and add the lime zest and juice with a couple of tbsp of the yogurt dressing. Tip in the squash, onions and chicken, add the chicory and toss everything together. Pile onto plates and drizzle with the remaining dressing. (If eating cold as a packed lunch, take the dressing in a pot and dress the salad when ready to eat.)

TIP Chicory is a naturally bitter vegetable, which stimulates the digestive juices. You will get more of the vitamin C, folate and beta-carotene content if you eat it raw.

BENEFITS low fat • calcium • fibre • vit c • iron • 4 of 5 a day • gluten free
PER SERVING 477 kcals • fat 13g • saturates 7g • carbs 42g • sugars 21g • fibre 13g • protein 41g • salt 1.4g

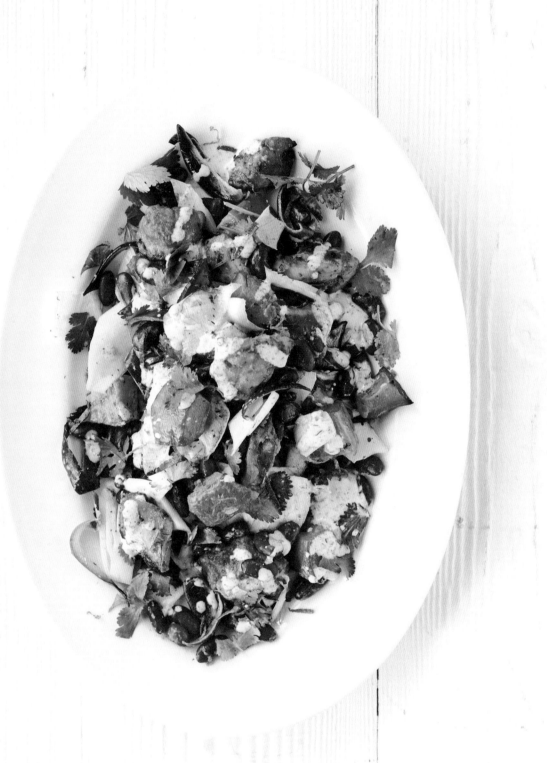

Pesto-crusted Cod with Puy Lentils

The homemade pesto on the cod creates a tasty crust as well as keeing the fish moist. You can use it on skinless chicken breasts too, but add an extra 10 mins or so to the cooking time.

Takes 25 mins   Serves 2

- large pack basil, leaves only
- 4 garlic cloves, 2 whole, 2 crushed
- 25g/1oz pine nuts
- 1 lemon
- 50ml/2fl oz olive oil
- 2 cod fillets
- 2 red chillies, finely chopped (deseeded if you don't like it too hot)
- 2 large tomatoes, roughly chopped
- 250g/9oz cooked Puy lentils

1 First, make the pesto. In a food processor, pulse the basil, whole garlic cloves, pine nuts, the juice of half the lemon and some seasoning, gradually adding most of the oil.
2 Heat oven to 180C/160C fan/ gas 4 and line a roasting tin with foil. Season the cod on both sides and coat each fillet in the pesto. Cook for 8-10 mins until a crust has formed and the cod is cooked through.
3 Meanwhile, heat the remaining oil in a small saucepan. Add the crushed garlic and the chillies, and cook for a couple of mins to release the flavour. Add the tomatoes and cook for 1 min more. Tip in the lentils, squeeze over the other half of the lemon, then season. Cook until piping hot and serve with the pesto cod.

TIP Puy lentils are rich in energising iron and molybdenum. Lentils also supply B vitamins, which help to regulate the nervous system and manage hormone levels.

BENEFITS fibre • vit c • iron • 2 of 5 a day • gluten free
PER SERVING 672 kcals • fat 37g • saturates 5g • carbs 34g • sugars 7g • fibre 11g • protein 45g • salt 1.6g

150 | The 7-day vitality plan

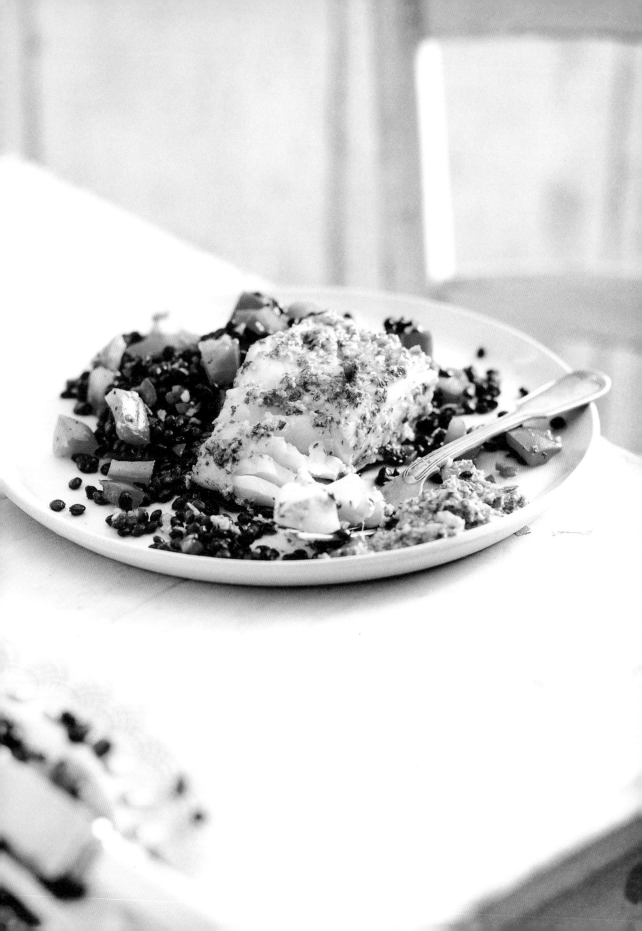

Smoked Paprika Paella with Cod & Peas

This is a delicious meal in one made with white fish and brown rice. Cod is an excellent source of stress-busting B vitamins and anti-anxiety magnesium.

🕐 Takes 55 mins   🥧 Serves 2

- 1 tbsp rapeseed oil
- 1 onion, finely chopped
- 2 garlic cloves, chopped
- 100g/4oz brown basmati rice
- 1 tsp turmeric
- 1 tsp smoked paprika
- 500ml/18fl oz reduced-salt vegetable bouillon
- 1 large red pepper, deseeded and chopped
- 1 large courgette, diced
- 125g/4½oz frozen peas
- 300g pack skinless Atlantic cod loins, cut into large chunks
- ⅓ small pack parsley, chopped
- ½ lemon, cut into wedges

1 Heat the oil in a non-stick frying pan over a medium-high heat and fry the onion and garlic for a couple of mins to soften. Add the rice and spices, stir briefly, then pour in the bouillon and add the pepper. Cover the pan, reduce the heat and leave to simmer for 20 mins. Stir in the courgette, cover and cook for 10 mins more.

2 Add the peas and cod, cover the pan and cook for 10 mins more until the rice is cooked and the liquid has been absorbed. Toss with the parsley and serve with lemon wedges.

BENEFITS low fat • low cal • folate • fibre • vit c • iron • 3 of 5 a day
PER SERVING 481 kcals • fat 9g • saturates 1g • carbs 55g • sugars 14g • fibre 11g • protein 38g • salt 0.4g

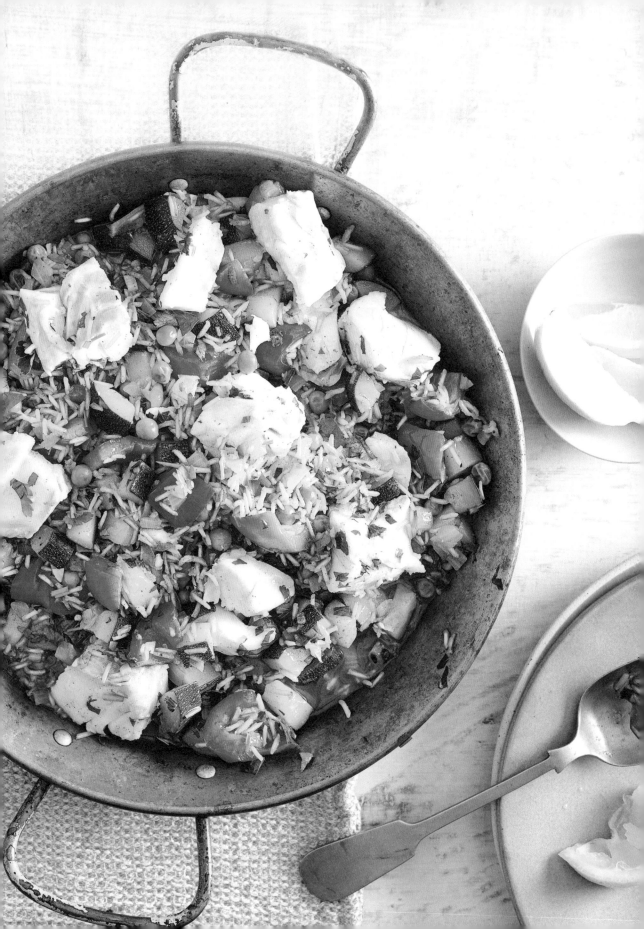

Lemon Sardines with Walnut & Pepper Dressing

Healthier fats such as fish oil work like an internal moisturiser, keeping skin hydrated and plumped up, while eating protein to produce collagen and elastin helps to keep skin strong and supple.

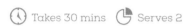 Takes 30 mins Serves 2

- 6 butterflied sardines, thawed if frozen
- 2 garlic cloves, finely grated
- juice and zest 1 lemon
- 2 tsp fresh oregano or I tsp soft thyme leaves, plus a few extra leaves for sprinkling
- 6 walnut halves
- 100g/4oz frozen sliced peppers (defrosted)
- small drizzle of rapeseed oil
- 175g/6oz baby spinach leaves
- the seeds from ½ pomegranate

1 Open up the sardines and smear the flesh with half the garlic, then grate over the lemon zest (reserving a little to serve) and season with black pepper. Scatter over half the herbs, then fold the fish in half to reshape them.

2 Put the walnuts, remaining herbs and the peppers in a bowl, then blitz to a rough purée with a stick blender. Add the remaining garlic and a generous squeeze of lemon from half of it then blitz again.

3 Rub a large non-stick frying pan with a little oil and heat a drop in a wok, then cook the sardines for 2 mins each side in the frying pan and quickly wilt the spinach in the wok. Arrange the spinach on 2 plates and top with the sardines, scatter over the pomegranate then top with the dressing. Sprinkle over the reserved lemon zest and a few herb leaves, then serve with the remaining half of the lemon, cut into wedges.

TIP Walnuts contain omega-3 fats, which improve the skin's elasticity. They're also a source of copper, a mineral that boosts collagen production.

BENEFITS low cal • omega-3 • calcium • folate • fibre • vit c • iron • 2 of 5 a day • gluten free
PER SERVING 333 kcals • fat 17g • saturates 3g • carbs 14g • sugars 12g • fibre 7g • protein 27g • salt 0.7g

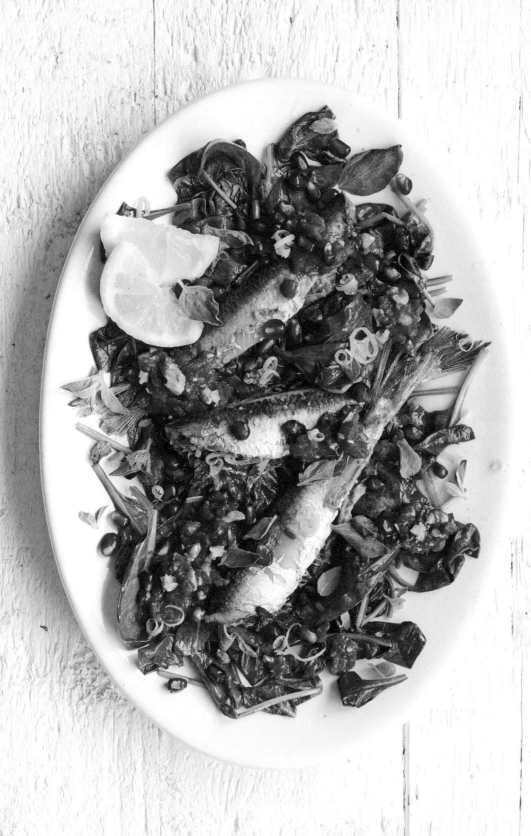

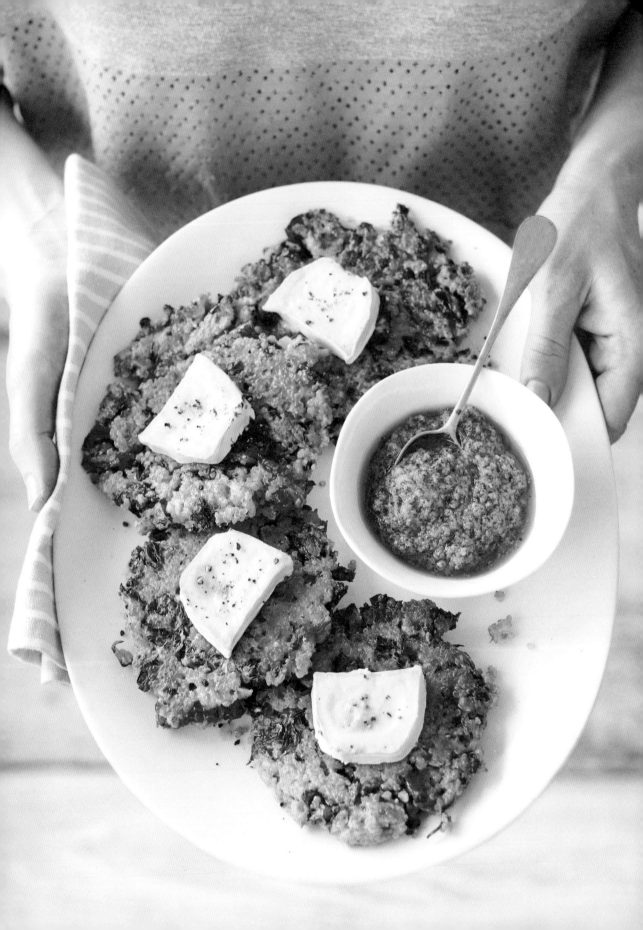

Chapter 3:

THE 7-DAY VEGETARIAN PLAN

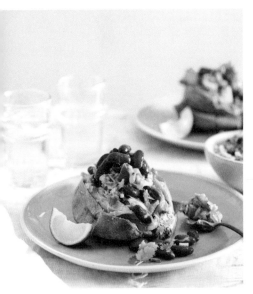
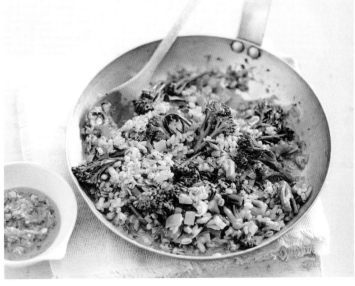
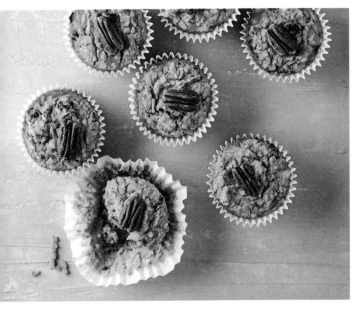
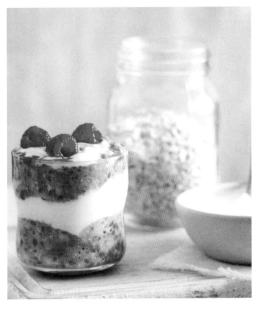

Enjoy the benefits of a vegetarian diet

The recipes forming this 7-day plan are lacto-ovo vegetarian, which means that the ingredients include plant-based foods as well as dairy and eggs. If you prefer to eat a vegan diet, we've included plenty of vegan recipes in the additional recipe section of this chapter. So whether you are a committed vegetarian or fancy a bit of an energising re-boot using fresh, vegetarian ingredients, this plan is for you.

A well-planned meat-free diet can have significant health benefits, ranging from a reduced risk of heart disease and bowel cancer to those who follow a vegetarian diet being less likely to be obese.

Gone are the days when, as a vegetarian, you had to rely on processed foods like textured vegetable protein (TVP) or manufactured quorn products, for your protein intake. There are plenty of natural, unprocessed plant sources like the quinoa in our Toasted sweetcorn, avocado & quinoa salad (page 210) or the chickpeas and nuts in our Burgers on page 216. As well as being important for repair and growth, protein helps to keep us full and satisfied and stabilises our energy levels. Making sure your meals are balanced in terms of protein and carbs will help you manage your cravings. We've used a broad range of plant-based protein sources in our recipe plan to ensure you obtain all the building blocks needed for good health and vitality.

As you flick through our recipes, you'll see that we use nuts and seeds, or their oils and butters, throughout. This is because they are a valuable source of omega-3 fatty acids – these are the essential fats that are vital for brain function and hormonal balance. Nuts and seeds supply the short chain version of these important fats, which our bodies must convert to the active long chain form (typically found in oily varieties of fish) – good plant sources include chia, flaxseeds, walnuts and almonds. Nuts and seeds are also full of the vitamins and minerals that non-vegetarians obtain from meat and fish – such as iron, zinc, magnesium and selenium.

Vegetarians are typically at an advantage to meat eaters when it comes to fibre and folate intake. Fibre helps keep the digestive system healthy, allows for a steady release of the energy from our food, while the soluble form from oats and flaxseeds helps us manage our cholesterol levels. We've used oats and flaxseeds in our Orange & blueberry bircher (page 164) – soaking or cooking oats helps to break down their natural phytate content so you can better access their nutrient goodness. Folate is a key vitamin for heart health and mood and is found in dark green leafy vegetables, nuts, seeds and beans – so in abundance in our vegetarian recipes!

If you follow a vegan diet it is important that you maintain your intake of calcium for strong healthy bones and teeth – sources include beans, nuts, seeds and green leafy veg. If you don't eat dairy or eggs, then you may be low in the vitamin B12. This vitamin is typically found in animal foods so look to include yeast extract, fortified versions of

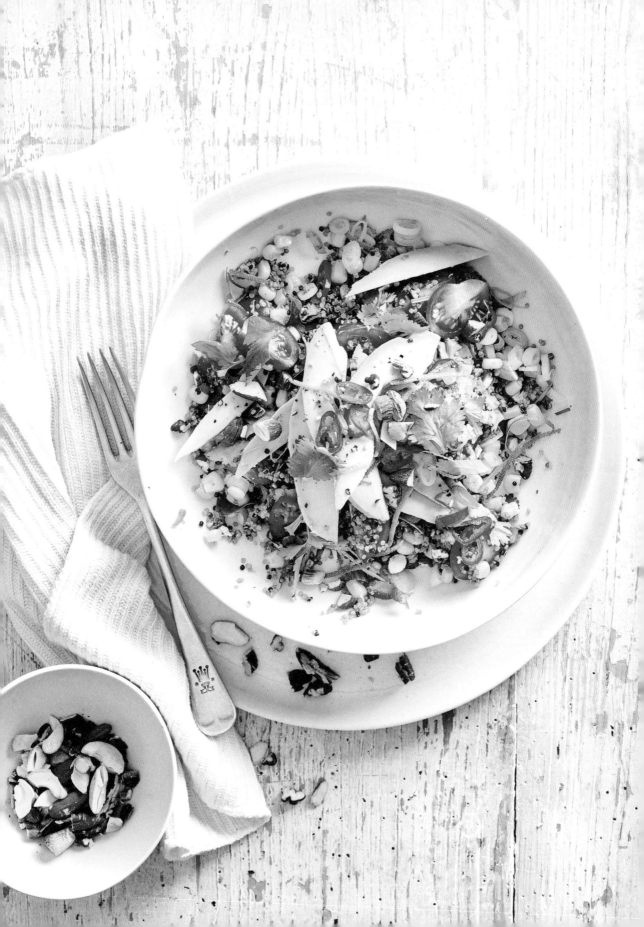

soya and cereals or consider taking a supplement.

Some believe it to be tricky to get enough iron from a meat-free diet – this needn't be the case. We've included recipes that combine vitamin C-rich foods, which aids our absorption of iron, with foods rich in this important energising mineral – try our Indian chickpeas with poached eggs (page 182) or Moroccan harira (page 200).

Once you've completed the 7 days you may wish to start to build your own vegetarian plan using the additional recipes in this chapter – all our recipes are packed with vegetarian ingredients bursting with vitamins, minerals and phytonutrients.

The secret to the success of any approach to healthy eating is preparation and planning, so we recommend using the Saturday before you start to do the shopping as well as a little bit of food prep.

We suggest you enjoy the meals as set out in the 7-day vegetarian chart for the most nutritionally balanced approach, but if you do want to mix, match or repeat dishes, you'll still get all the benefits of eating unprocessed and wholesome foods.

THE 7-DAY VEGETARIAN PLAN (Serves 2)

	BREAKFAST	LUNCH	DINNER
Sunday	Almond crêpes with avocado & nectarines	Green rice with beetroot & apple salsa	Moroccan harira
Monday	Berry bircher	Lemon roast vegetables with yogurt tahini & pomegranate	Lentil ragu with courgetti
Tuesday	Basil scramble with wilted spinach & seared tomatoes	Summer carrot, tarragon & white bean soup	Sweet potato jackets with guacamole & kidney beans
Wednesday	Orange & blueberry bircher	Feta frittatas with carrot & celery salad	Lentil ragu with courgetti
Thursday	Berry bircher	Moroccan harira	Niçoise egg salad
Friday	Orange & blueberry bircher	Indian chickpeas with poached eggs	End-of-the-week noodles with ginger & tamari
Saturday	Berry bircher	Summer carrot, tarragon & white bean soup	Barley & broccoli risotto with lemon & basil

Almond Crêpes
with Avocado & Nectarines

These simple crêpes will keep you going all morning, yet they're gluten-free and low in carbs. Pomegranate seeds don't just add an extra visual flourish, they contain protective antioxidants including vitamin C.

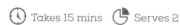 Takes 15 mins   Serves 2

- 2 large eggs
- 3 tbsp ground almonds
- 2 tsp rapeseed oil
- 1 avocado, halved, stoned and flesh lightly crushed
- 2 ripe nectarines, stoned and sliced
- seeds from ½ pomegranate
- ½ lime, cut into 2 wedges, for squeezing over

1 Beat 1 egg and 1½ tbsp of the almonds in a small bowl with 1 tbsp water. Heat 1 tsp oil in a large non-stick frying pan over a medium heat and pour in the egg mixture, swirling the pan to evenly cover the base. Cook until the mixture sets and turns golden on the underside, about 2 mins. (There is no need to flip it over.) Turn it out onto a plate and make another one with 1 tbsp water, the remaining egg, oil and almonds.

2 Top each crêpe with the avocado, nectarines and pomegranate, and squeeze over the lime at the table.

BENEFITS vegetarian • fibre • vit c • 2 of 5 a day, gluten free
PER SERVING 457 kcals • fat 34g • saturates 5g • carbs 18g • sugars 16g • fibre 7g • protein 16g • salt 0.2g

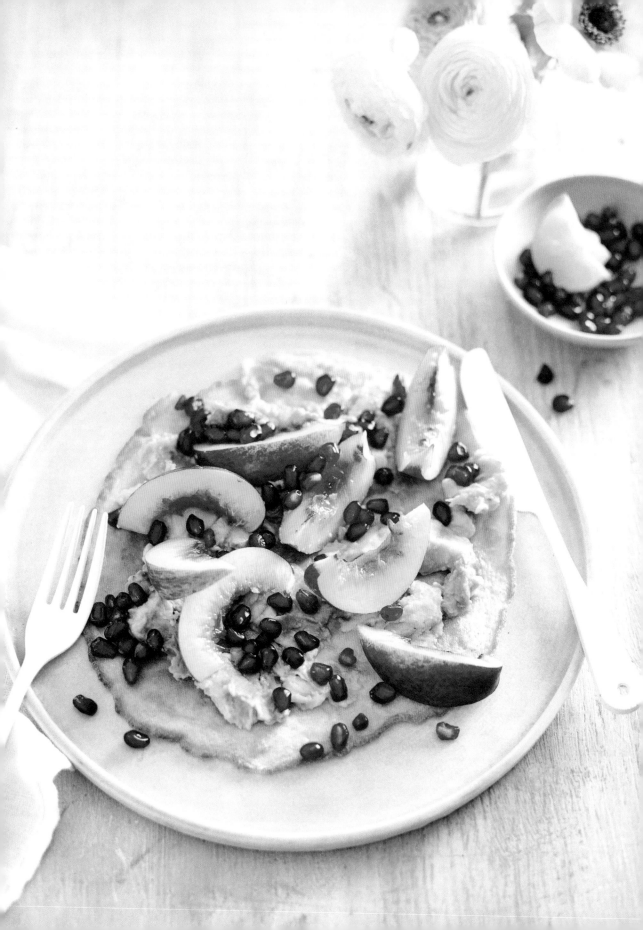

Orange & Blueberry Bircher

Citrus fruits like oranges are rich in collagen-supportive vitamin C, and are great for promoting skin health and elasticity. Make double and keep in the fridge, then enjoy on Friday too.

🕐 Takes 10 mins, plus overnight soaking   ◧ Serves 2

- 75g/3oz porridge oats
- 2 tbsp golden flaxseeds
- finely grated zest of ½ orange, plus 2 oranges, peeled and chopped
- 175g/6oz live bio yogurt
- 4 handfuls blueberries from a 150g pack

1 Mix the oats and flaxseeds with the orange zest. Pour over 300ml/½ pint boiling water and leave overnight. The next day, stir in three-quarters of the yogurt, spoon into glasses or bowls, top with the chopped oranges, the remaining yogurt and blueberries.

TIP Oats are a good source of silica for strong, lustrous hair.

BENEFITS vegetarian • low fat • calcium • folate • fibre • vit c • 2 of 5 a day
PER SERVING 345 kcals • fat 9g •saturates 3g • carbs 48g • sugars 22g • fibre 8g • protein 13g • salt 0.2g

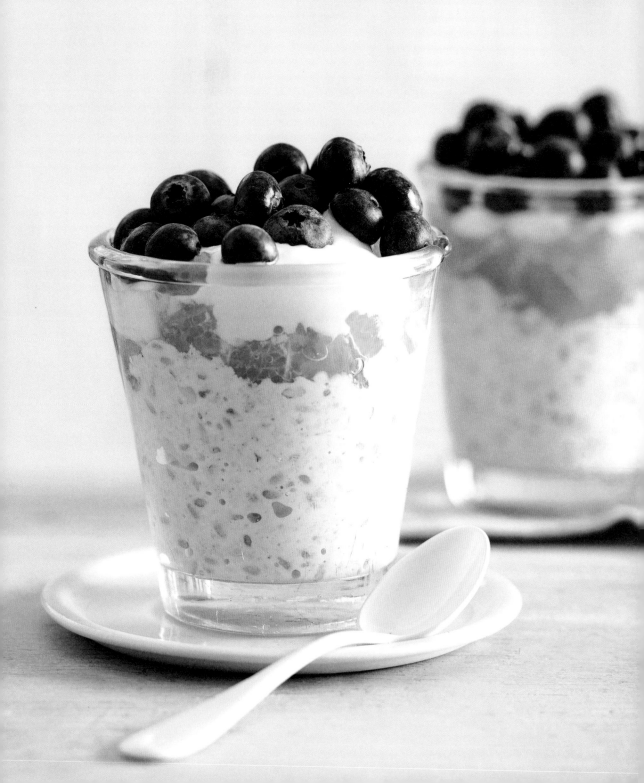

Berry Bircher

Soaking oats and seeds overnight makes them easier to digest. This, consumed with fruit, adds up to a fabulously nutritious start to the day with all the right kinds of fats, fibre, vitamins and minerals.

Takes 10 mins, plus overnight chilling   Serves 2

- 75g/3oz porridge oats
- 2 tbsp golden linseeds
- 2 ripe bananas
- 140g/5oz frozen raspberries
- 175g/6oz live bio yogurt

1 Tip the oats and seeds into a bowl, and pour over 200ml/7fl oz boiling water and stir well. Add the bananas and three-quarters of the raspberries (chill the remainder), mash together, then cover and chill overnight.

2 The next day, layer the raspberry oats in 2 tumblers or bowls with the yogurt, top with the reserved raspberries and serve.

BENEFITS *vegetarian • low fat • calcium • folate • fibre • vit c • 2 of 5 a day*
PER SERVING *372 kcals • fat 9g • saturates 2g • carbs 55g • sugars 27g • fibre 9g • protein 13g • salt 0.2g*

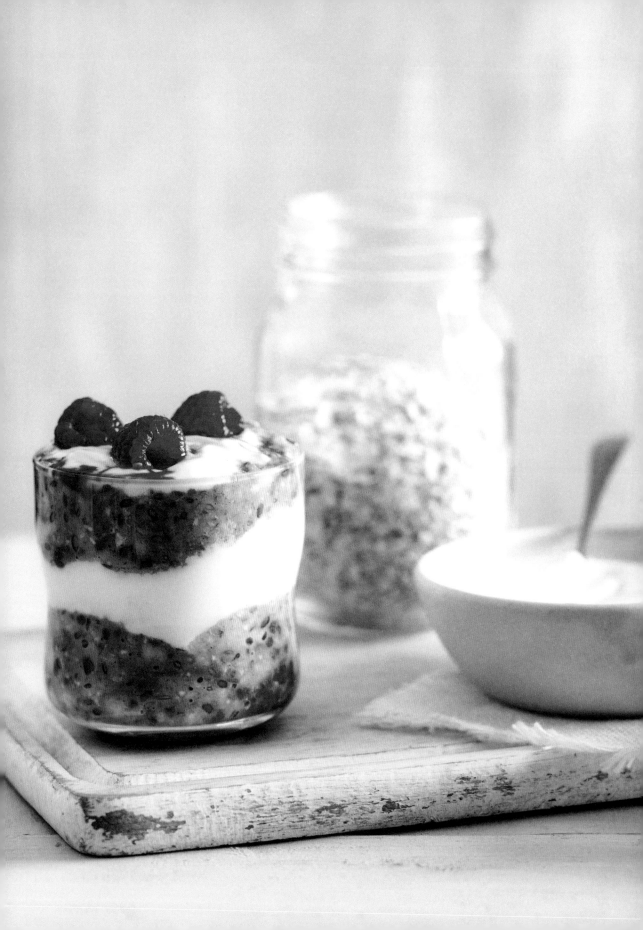

Basil Scramble with Wilted Spinach & Seared Tomatoes

Forget toast and serve our scramble with tomatoes and spinach for a speedy supercharged breakfast. A true superfood, spinach is bursting with nutrients that are important for our skin, hair and bone health.

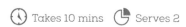 Takes 10 mins Serves 2

- 1 tbsp rapeseed oil, plus 1 tsp
- 3 tomatoes, halved
- 4 large eggs
- 4 tbsp live bio yogurt
- ⅓ small pack basil, chopped
- 175g pack baby spinach, dried well (if it needs washing)

1 Heat 1 tsp oil in a large non-stick frying pan, add the tomatoes and cook, cut-side down, over a medium heat. While they are cooking, beat the eggs in a jug with the yogurt, 2 tbsp water, plenty of black pepper and the basil.

2 Transfer the tomatoes to serving plates. Add the spinach to the pan and wilt, stirring a few times, while you cook the eggs.

3 Heat the rest of the oil in a non-stick pan over a medium heat, pour in the egg mixture and stir every now and then until scrambled and just set. Spoon the spinach onto the plates and top with the scrambled eggs.

BENEFITS *vegetarian • calcium • folate • vit c • 2 of 5 a day • gluten free*
PER SERVING *297 kcals • fat 19g • saturates 5g • carbs 10g • sugars 10g • fibre 2g • protein 20g • salt 0.6g*

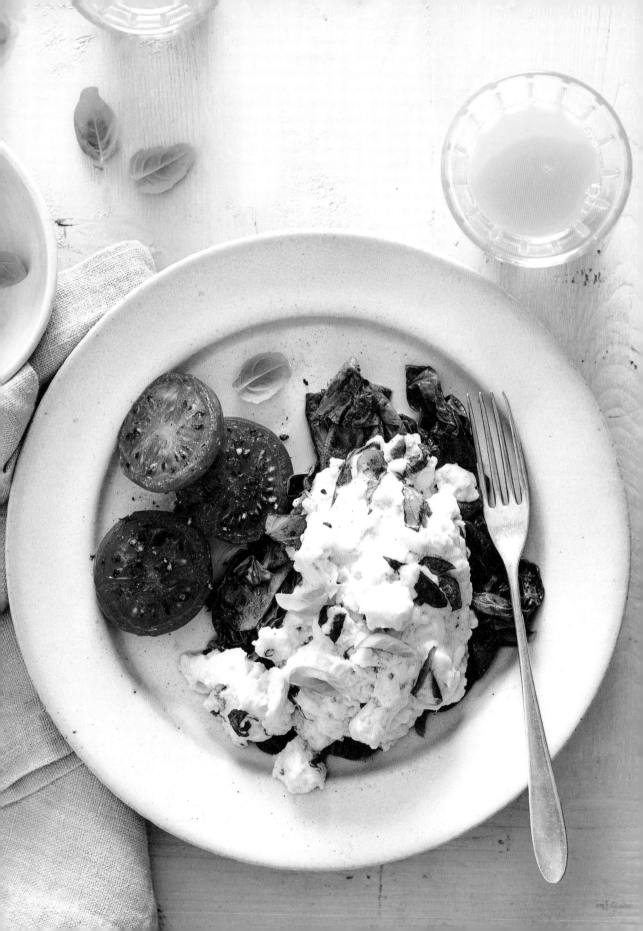

Breakfast Muffins

These good-for-you muffins, based on the flavours of carrot cake, taste delicious, and have a surprise ingredient – beans! Don't let that put you off as they don't just add to your 5 a day, they provide a lovely moist texture. Enjoy them with a cup of refreshing green tea, which is full of antioxidants.

🕐 Takes 30 mins　　🥧 Makes 8

- 400g can cannellini beans in water, drained
- 1 tsp ground cinnamon
- 50g/2oz porridge oats
- 2 large eggs
- 1 tbsp rapeseed oil
- 2 tbsp maple syrup
- 1 tsp vanilla extract
- grated zest small orange
- 85g/3oz coarsely grated carrot
- 50g/2oz raisins
- 40g/1½oz pecans, 8 halves reserved then rest roughly broken
- 1 tsp baking powder

1 Heat oven to 180C/160C fan/gas 4 and line a 12-hole muffin tin with 8 paper cases. Tip the drained beans into a bowl then add the cinnamon, oats, eggs, rapeseed oil, maple syrup, vanilla extract and orange zest. Blitz with a stick blender until really smooth so the beans and oats have ground down as much as possible.

2 Stir in the grated carrot, raisins, chopped pecans and baking powder, stir well, then spoon into the muffin cases. If you have a large ice cream scoop, use that to get nice even ones.

3 Top each muffin with a reserved nut then bake for 20 mins until set and light brown. Cool on a wire wrack. They will keep in the fridge for a couple of days or will freeze for 6 weeks. Thaw at room temperature.

BENEFITS vegetarian
PER MUFFIN 156 kcals • fat 7g • saturates 1g • carbs 16g • sugars 8g • fibre 4g • protein 5g • salt 0.2g

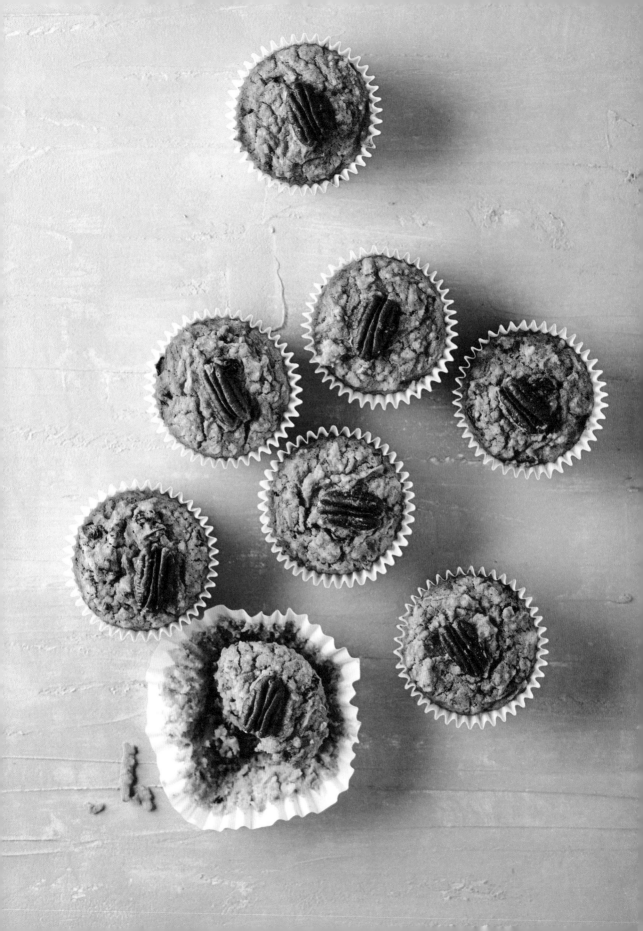

One-pan Summer Eggs

Satisfy your hunger with this fresh and easy vegetarian breakfast, or brunch if you prefer.

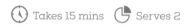 Takes 15 mins   Serves 2

- 1 tbsp olive oil
- 400g/14oz courgettes, cut into chunks
- 200g/7oz cherry tomatoes, halved
- 1 garlic clove, crushed
- 2 eggs
- few basil leaves

1 Heat the oil in a non-stick frying pan, then add the courgettes. Fry for 5 mins, stirring every so often until they start to soften, add the tomatoes and garlic, then cook for a few mins more. Stir in a little seasoning, then make 2 gaps in the mix and crack in the eggs. Cover the pan with a lid or a sheet of foil, then cook for 2-3 mins until the eggs are done to your liking. Scatter over a few basil leaves and serve with crusty bread.

BENEFITS *vegetarian • low cal • vit C • folate • 2 of 5 a day • gluten free*
PER SERVING *196 kcals • fat 13g • saturates 3g • carbs 7g • sugars 6g • fibre 3g • protein 12g • salt 0.25g*

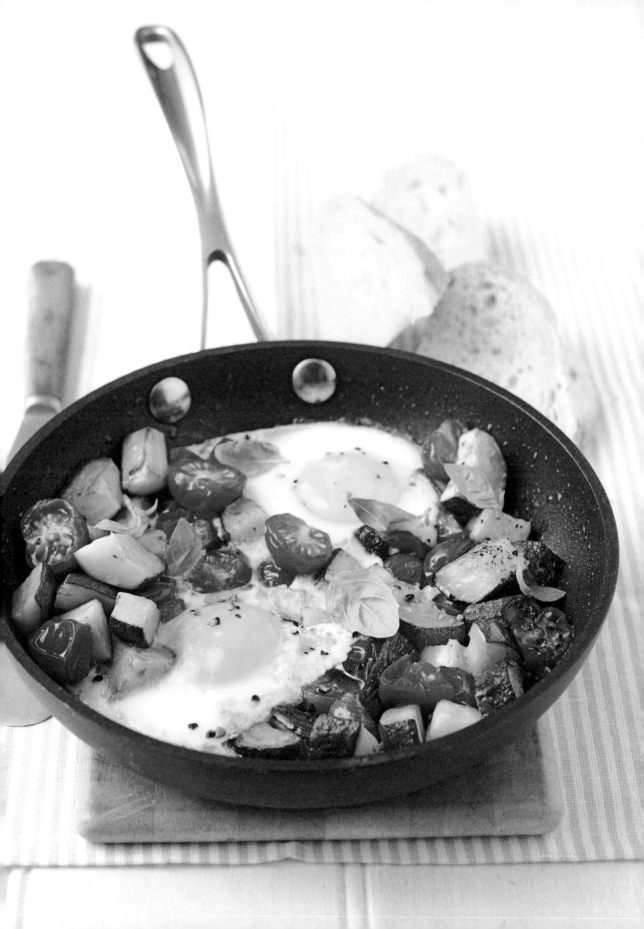

Feta Frittatas with Carrot & Celery Salad

Combining carrots with foods naturally rich in fats, like eggs and cheese, helps us to absorb vitamin A.

 Takes 40 mins 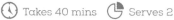 Serves 2

FOR THE FRITTATAS
- 2 tsp rapeseed oil, plus a drizzle for the salad (optional)
- 1 large leek, well washed and thinly sliced
- 25g/1oz baby spinach
- 3 large eggs
- ⅓ pack dill, stalks removed, fronds chopped
- 2 tbsp live bio yogurt
- 50g/2oz feta, crumbled
- 1 garlic clove, finely grated

FOR THE SALAD
- 2 tsp balsamic vinegar
- 2 tsp tahini
- 2 celery sticks, sliced
- 2 carrots, peeled into ribbons
- 1 very small red onion, thinly sliced
- 2 romaine lettuce leaves, torn into pieces
- 6 pitted Kalamata olives, rinsed

1 Heat oven to 220C/200C fan/gas 7 with a muffin tin inside. Heat the oil in a frying pan and fry the leek for about 4 mins, stirring regularly, over a medium-high heat to soften it. Stir in the spinach and cook for 1 min until wilted down, then set aside to cool slightly.

2 Beat the eggs, dill, yogurt and feta together in a jug with black pepper and the garlic. Add the leeks and spinach, and stir well. Take the muffin tin out of the oven and drop in 4 muffin cases, add the egg mixture and bake for 15-18 mins until set and golden.

3 Meanwhile, mix the balsamic vinegar with the tahini and 1-2 tbsp water in a bowl to make a dressing, then toss with the vegetables and olives. Pile onto plates, carefully remove the paper cases from the frittatas and serve.

4 These will keep for 2 days in the fridge. If you're packing this for a work lunch, take the salad and dressing in separate containers.

TIP Spinach is rich in lutein, good for eye health.

BENEFITS vegetarian • calcium • folate • fibre • vit c • iron • 3 of 5 a day • gluten free
PER SERVING 378 kcals • fat 22g • saturates 7g • carbs 18g • sugars 15g • fibre 12g • protein 21g • salt 1.4g

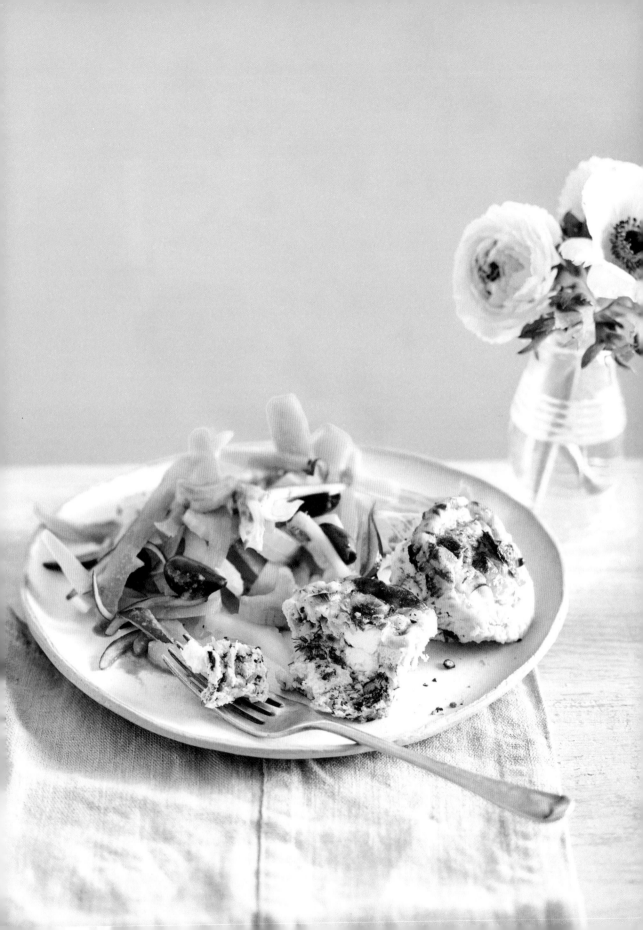

Lemon Roast Vegetables with Yogurt Tahini & Pomegranate

Savoury yogurt has become really popular and we've used tahini in our version, which is a great way to top up levels of calcium, iron, zinc and magnesium. It's naturally high in fats – the majority of which are heart-friendly.

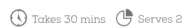 Takes 30 mins   Serves 2

- 1 red pepper, deseeded and chopped
- 1 aubergine, diced
- 1 red onion, halved and thinly sliced
- 1 unwaxed lemon, ¼ finely chopped (skin and all), the rest juiced
- 1 tbsp rapeseed oil, plus extra to drizzle (optional)
- 400g can chickpeas in water, drained
- 1 garlic clove
- 2 tbsp tahini
- 3 tbsp natural bio yogurt
- seeds from ½ pomegranate
- ⅓ small pack parsley or coriander, chopped

1 Heat oven to 240C/220C fan/gas 7. Put the vegetables and chopped lemon in a large flameproof roasting tin and drizzle with 1 tbsp oil. Massage into the veg so they are all well coated, then put the tin on the hob and fry, stirring, for 5 mins until starting to char. Stir in 2 handfuls of the chickpeas, and roast in the oven for 15 mins.

2 Put the rest of the chickpeas in a bowl with the garlic, tahini, yogurt, lemon juice and 3 tbsp water, and blitz with a stick blender until really smooth and thick.

3 Spoon the yogurt tahini onto 2 plates and top with the roasted veg, pomegranate seeds and parsley. Season with black pepper and a drizzle of extra oil, if you like. Save time and make this the night before. If you're taking it for a packed lunch, just layer the yogurt and veg in containers and keep in the fridge.

BENEFITS *vegetarian • calcium • iron • folate • fibre • vit c • 4 of 5 a day • gluten free*
PER SERVING 513 kcals • fat 24g • saturates 4g • carbs 42g • sugars 22g • fibre 21g • protein 20g • salt 0.2g

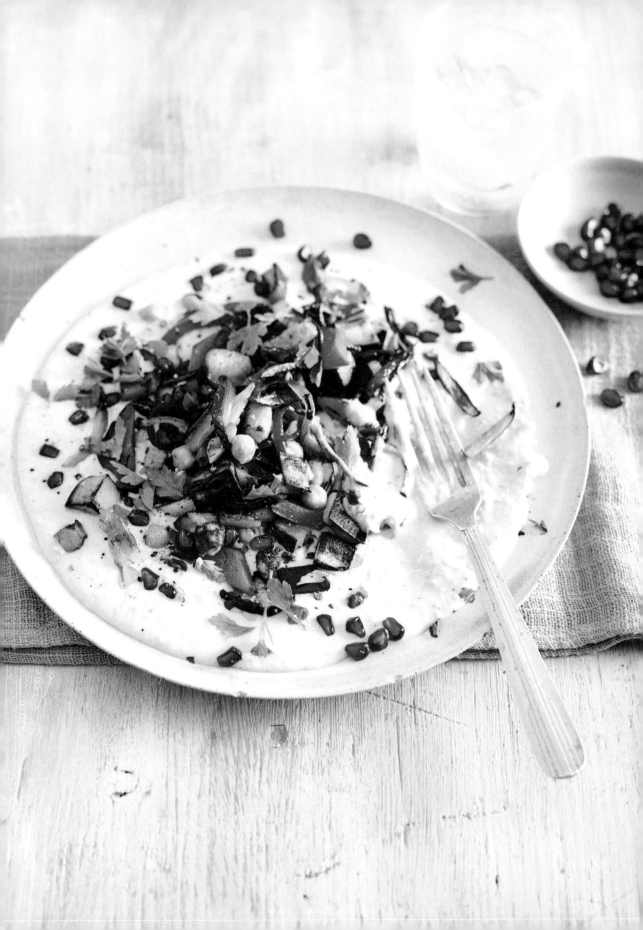

Summer Carrot, Tarragon & White Bean Soup

A bowl of this soup will supply your body with the fibre needed for a healthy gut. Eat half and enjoy on 2 days as part of this veggie plan.

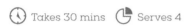 Takes 30 mins   Serves 4

- 1 tbsp rapeseed oil
- 2 large leeks, well washed, halved lengthways and finely sliced
- 700g/1lb 9oz carrots, chopped
- 1.4 litres/2½ pints hot reduced-salt vegetable bouillon
- 4 garlic cloves, finely grated
- 2 x 400g cans cannellini beans
- ⅔ small pack tarragon, leaves roughly chopped

1 Heat the oil over a medium heat in a large pan and fry the leeks and carrots for 5 mins to soften.
2 Pour over the stock, stir in the garlic, the beans with their liquid, and three-quarters of the tarragon, then cover and simmer for 15 mins or until the veg is just tender. Stir in the remaining tarragon before serving.

TIP Carrots are a good source of carotenoids, which help to prevent the oxidative damage associated with aging.

BENEFITS vegetarian • low fat • folate • fibre • 3 of 5 a day
PER SERVING 271 kcals • fat 6g • saturates 1g • carbs 38g • sugars 17g • fibre 13g • protein 11g • salt 0.7g

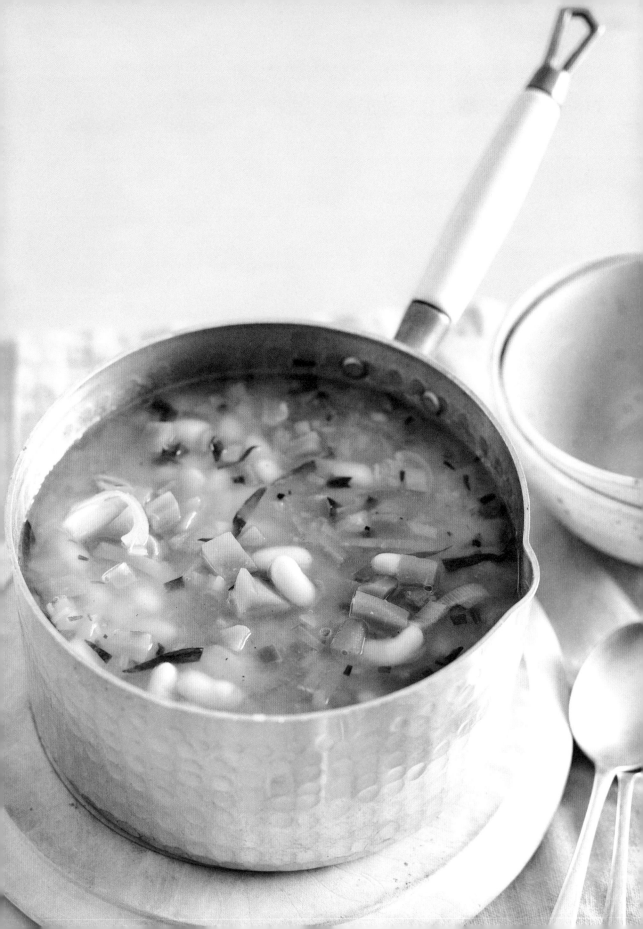

Green Rice with Beetroot & Apple Salsa

We've included walnuts in our salsa because they're rich in essential omega-3 fats, which are important for the heart, healthy hormones, brain function and mood. We took them from a bag of mixed nuts and used the rest for Friday's noodle dish.

 Takes 35 mins   Serves 2

FOR THE RICE
- 85g/3oz brown basmati rice
- 140g/5oz fine green beans
- ½ small cucumber, finely diced
- ½ bunch spring onions (about 5), sliced
- ⅓ pack mint, chopped, plus extra leaves to serve
- juice ½ lemon

FOR THE SALSA
- 1 cooked beetroot, diced
- 1 small apple, cored and diced
- 1 small red onion, finely chopped
- 25g/1oz walnut halves, roughly broken
- 1 tbsp balsamic vinegar

1 Boil the rice for 20 mins, then add the green beans and cook 5 mins more until both are just tender. Drain and leave to cool slightly before stirring in the cucumber, spring onions, mint and lemon juice.
2 Meanwhile, stir all the salsa ingredients together.
3 Spoon the rice onto plates and serve with the salsa, scattered with a few extra mint leaves.

BENEFITS vegan • low fat • low cal • folate • fibre • 3 of 5 a day • gluten free
PER SERVING 332 kcals • fat 11g • saturates 1g • carbs 45g • sugars 12g • fibre 8g • protein 10g • salt 0.1g

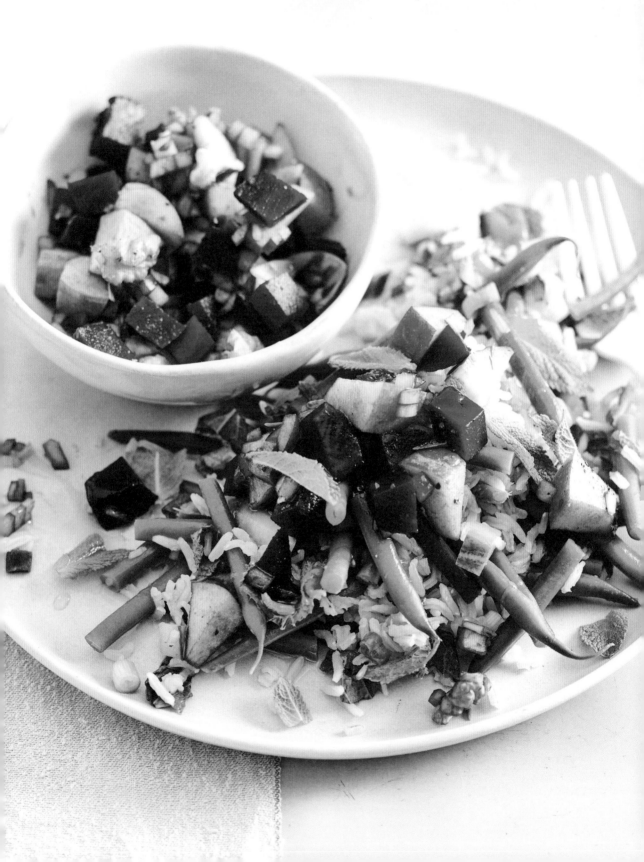

Indian Chickpeas with Poached Eggs

The chickpeas in this spicy lunch are a good source of manganese, which we need for healthy bone structure. Their fibre helps regulate cholesterol, manage appetite and reduce food cravings too.

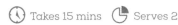 Takes 15 mins Serves 2

- 1 tbsp rapeseed oil
- 2 garlic cloves, chopped
- 1 yellow pepper, deseeded and diced
- ½-1 red chilli, deseeded and chopped
- ½ bunch spring onions (about 5), tops and whites sliced but kept separate
- 1 tsp ground cumin, plus a little extra to serve (optional)
- 1 tsp ground coriander
- ½ tsp turmeric
- 3 tomatoes, cut into wedges
- ⅓ pack coriander, chopped
- 400g can chickpeas in water, drained but liquid reserved
- ½ tsp reduced-salt bouillon powder
- 4 large eggs

1 Heat the oil in a non-stick sauté pan, add the garlic, pepper, chilli and the whites from the spring onions, and fry for 5 mins over a medium-high heat. Meanwhile, put a large pan of water on to boil.

2 Add the spices, tomatoes, most of the chopped coriander and the chickpeas to the sauté pan and cook for 1-2 mins more. Stir in the bouillon powder and enough liquid from the chickpeas to moisten everything, then leave to simmer gently.

3 Once the water is at a rolling boil, crack in your eggs and poach for 2 mins, then remove with a slotted spoon. Stir the spring onion tops into the chickpeas, then very lightly crush a few of the chickpeas with a fork or potato masher. Spoon the chickpea mixture onto plates, scatter with the reserved coriander and top with the eggs. Serve with an extra sprinkle of cumin, if you like.

BENEFITS vegetarian • low cal • folate • fibre • vit c • iron • 3 of 5 a day
PER SERVING 412 kcals • fat 20g • saturates 4g • carbs 27g • sugars 8g • fibre 10g • protein 24g • salt 0.3g

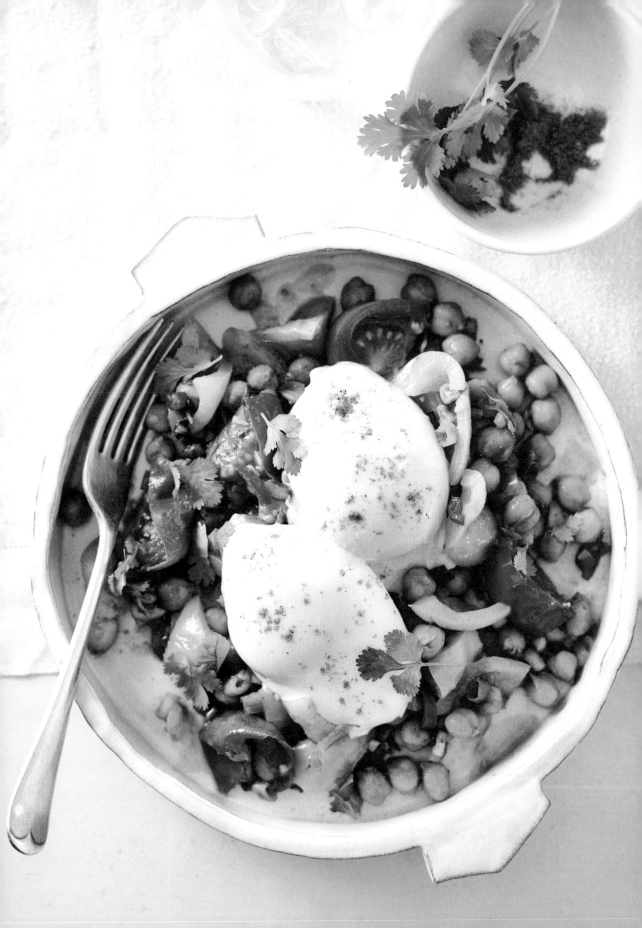

Grilled Aubergine Tabbouleh

This is a vegan tabbouleh with all the flavours of summer. The coconut and tahini dressing adds a creamy, nutty element to this winning couscous.

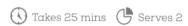 Takes 25 mins   Serves 2

- 2 tbsp rapeseed oil
- 1 large aubergine, diced
- 160g/5½oz wholegrain couscous
- ½ cucumber, diced
- 200g/7oz cherry tomatoes, halved
- small pack mint, roughly chopped
- small pack parsley, roughly chopped

FOR THE DRESSING
- juice 1 lemon
- 5 tbsp coconut yogurt
- 2 tbsp tahini
- 1 tbsp maple syrup

1 Heat the rapeseed oil in a frying pan over a medium-high heat and add the aubergine. Cook for 10 mins until soft and cooked through.
2 Meanwhile, put the couscous in a large bowl and pour over 200ml/7fl oz boiling water. Cover with cling film and leave to stand for 5-6 mins. Combine all the ingredients for the dressing and season to taste.
3 When the couscous has absorbed all the water, mix it up with a fork. Season and stir in the cucumber, tomatoes and herbs. Add half the dressing and toss to coat. Scatter over the aubergine and serve with the rest of the dressing.

TIP Mint is excellent for digestion, especially in the form of mint tea. Simply pour boiling water over fresh sprigs of mint.

BENEFITS vegan • calcium • folate • fibre • vit c • iron • 3 of 5 a day
PER SERVING 630 kcals • fat 33g • saturates 10g • carbs 58g • sugars 18g • fibre 14g • protein 17g • salt 0.1g

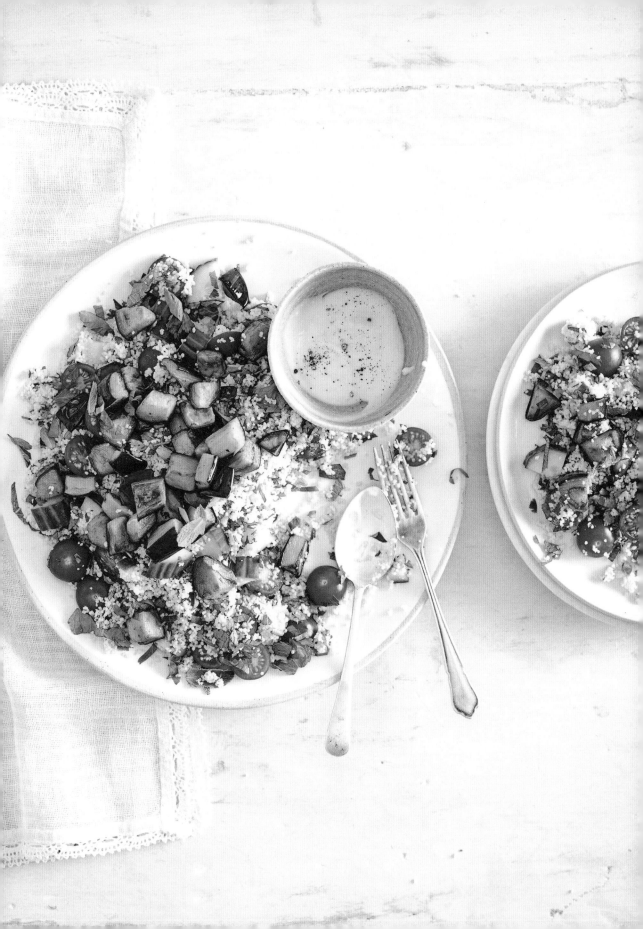

Masala Frittata with Avocado Salsa

This serves four so eat it warm with salad one day and cold the next. Alternatively, just use a smaller pan and halve the ingredients

⏱ Takes 40 mins ◔ Serves 4

- 2 tbsp rapeseed oil
- 3 onions, 2½ thinly sliced, ½ finely chopped
- 1 tbsp medium curry powder
- 500g/1lb 2oz cherry tomatoes, halved
- 1 red chilli, deseeded and finely chopped
- small pack coriander, roughly chopped
- 8 large eggs, beaten
- 1 avocado, stoned, peeled and cubed
- juice 1 lemon

1 Heat the oil in a medium non-stick, ovenproof frying pan. Tip in the sliced onions and cook over a medium heat for about 10 mins until soft and golden. Add the curry powder and fry for 1 min more, then tip in half the tomatoes and half the chilli. Cook until the mixture is thick and the tomatoes have all burst.

2 Heat the grill to high. Add half the coriander to the eggs and season, then pour over the spicy onion mixture. Stir gently once or twice, then cook over a low heat for 8-10 mins until almost set. Transfer to the grill for 3-5 mins until set.

3 To make the salsa, mix the avocado, remaining chilli and tomatoes, chopped onion, remaining chopped coriander and the lemon juice together, then season and serve with the frittata.

BENEFITS vegetarian • low cal • vit C • folate • 2 of 5 a day
PER SERVING 320 kcals • fat 22g • saturates 4g • carbs 12g • sugars 9g • fibre 5g • protein 15g • salt 0.5g

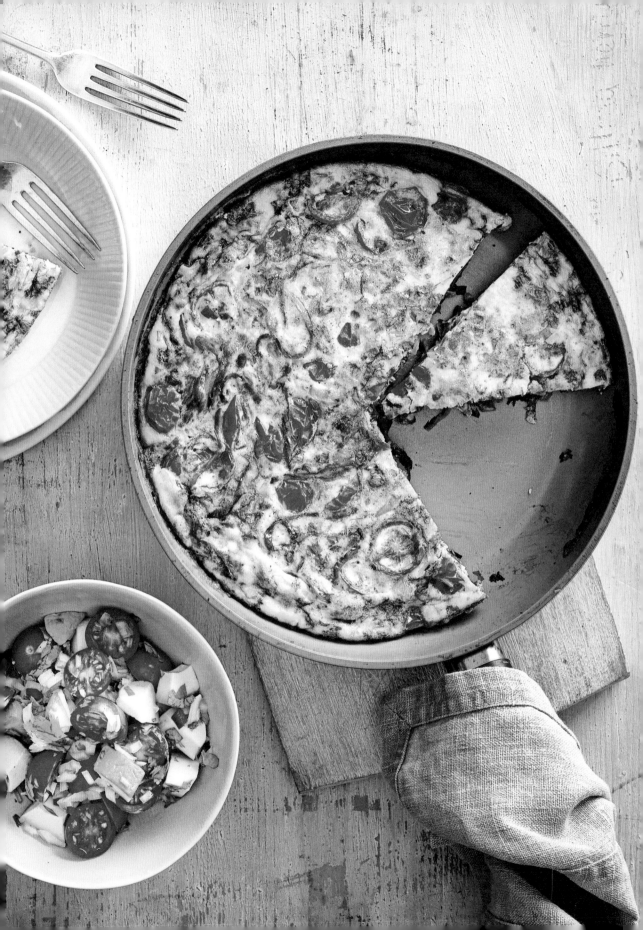

Kale & Quinoa Patties

Quick and easy to prepare, these are perfect for lunch, or serve with a green salad for a light dinner.

⏱ Takes 1 hour 5 mins ◔ Serves 4 (easily halved)

- 140g/5oz quinoa
- 500ml/18fl oz hot vegetable bouillon
- 100g/4oz kale, stalks removed, leaves roughly chopped
- 3 tbsp olive oil
- 1 small onion, finely chopped
- 2 garlic cloves, crushed
- 75g/2½oz fresh white breadcrumbs
- 2 medium eggs, beaten
- 50g/2oz sundried tomatoes, roughly chopped
- 100g/4oz goat's cheese, cut from a round log
- green salad, to serve (optional)

FOR THE PESTO
- ½ small pack basil, leaves only
- ½ small pack parsley, leaves only
- 2 garlic cloves, crushed
- 50g/2oz pine nuts, toasted
- 50g/2oz Parmesan, grated
- 150ml/1/4pt olive oil
- juice 1 lemon

1 Put the quinoa in a saucepan and pour over the hot stock. Simmer for 18-20 mins over a gentle heat until the grains have puffed up and the liquid has disappeared. Remove from the heat and allow to cool. Meanwhile, bring a large saucepan of water to the boil. Add the kale and simmer for 6-8 mins until cooked through. Drain, squeeze out any excess water and set aside.

2 Put 1 tbsp olive oil in a small frying pan over a medium heat. Add the onion and cook for 2-3 mins until translucent. Add the garlic and cook for 1 min more. Tip the cooked quinoa into a bowl and add the kale, onion, garlic, breadcrumbs, egg and sundried tomatoes. Season well and mix to combine. Set aside.

3 To make the pesto, put the basil, parsley, garlic, pine nuts and Parmesan in a small food processor. Pulse, slowly pouring in the oil, until you have a thick pesto. Squeeze in the lemon juice to loosen, then set aside.

4 Gently heat 2 tbsp olive oil in a shallow frying pan. Using your hands, form the quinoa mixture into 8 round patties. Add to the frying pan and fry for 4-5 mins each side until crisp and golden.

5 Heat the grill to high and put a slice of goat's cheese on top of each patty. Place under the grill to brown and melt the cheese slightly – this will take a matter of seconds, so keep an eye on them. Top each patty with a generous spoonful of pesto and serve with some fresh green leaves, if you like.

TIP Kale provides powerful antioxidants, like vitamin C, and damage-reducing sulforaphane.

BENEFITS vegetarian • vit c • iron • 1 of 5 a day
PER SERVING 564 kcals • fat 33g • saturates 9g • carbs 43g • sugars 9g • fibre 3g • protein 21g • salt 1.4g

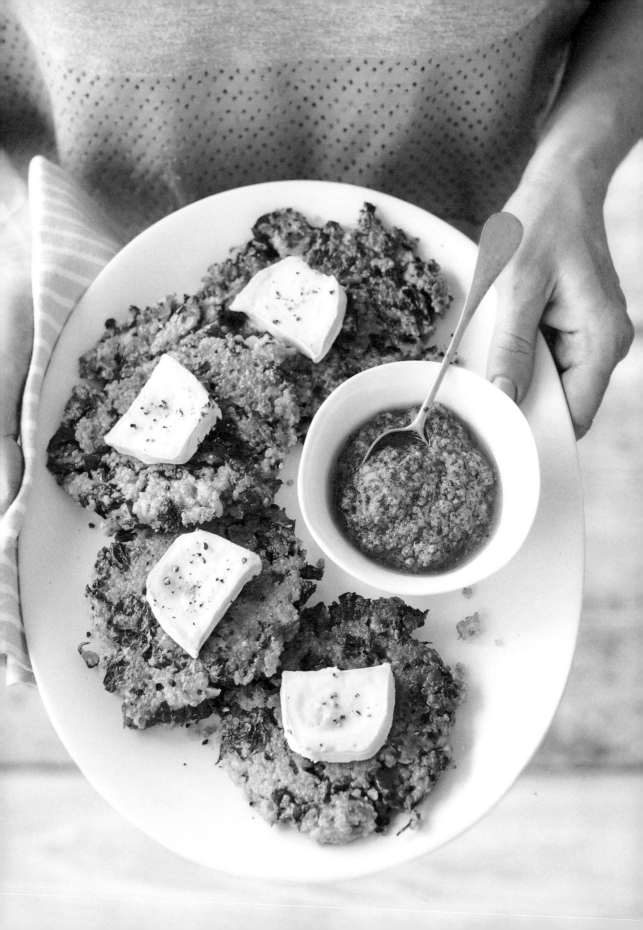

Baked Potatoes with Spicy Dhal

Curcumin in turmeric is thought to fight age-related decline and here it's added to a spicy lentil dhal to serve on fluffy jacket potatoes. It's delicious on brown rice too.

Takes 1 hour 10 mins   SERVES 2

- 2 baking potatoes (Vivaldi have a lovely creamy texture)
- 1 tbsp rapeseed oil
- ½ tsp each cumin seeds, black mustard seeds and ground turmeric
- 1 onion, thinly sliced
- 3 garlic cloves, sliced
- 1 red chilli, deseeded and sliced
- 85g/3oz red split lentils
- 1 tomato, chopped
- 400ml/14fl oz vegetable bouillon
- 210g can chickpeas, drained and rinsed
- good handful chopped coriander leaves

1 Heat oven to 200C/180C fan/gas 6. Put the potatoes in the oven and bake for 1 hour until tender and the skin is crispy.
2 While the potatoes are baking, make the dhal. Heat the oil in a medium pan and fry the spices to release their flavours. As soon as they start to crackle, tip in the onion, garlic and chilli, with a splash of water to stop the spices from burning. Cook for 5 mins until the onion softens.
3 Add the lentils, tomato and stock, then cover and cook for 10 mins. Tip in the chickpeas, cover and cook for 10 mins more until the lentils are tender. Season the dhal to taste, stir in the coriander and spoon on to the jacket potatoes.

BENEFITS *vegetarian • low fat • folate • vit c • iron • 2 of 5 a day • fibre*
PER SERVING *556 kcals • fat 8g • saturates 1g • carbs 96g • sugar 10g • fibre 12g • protein 23g • salt 1.1g*

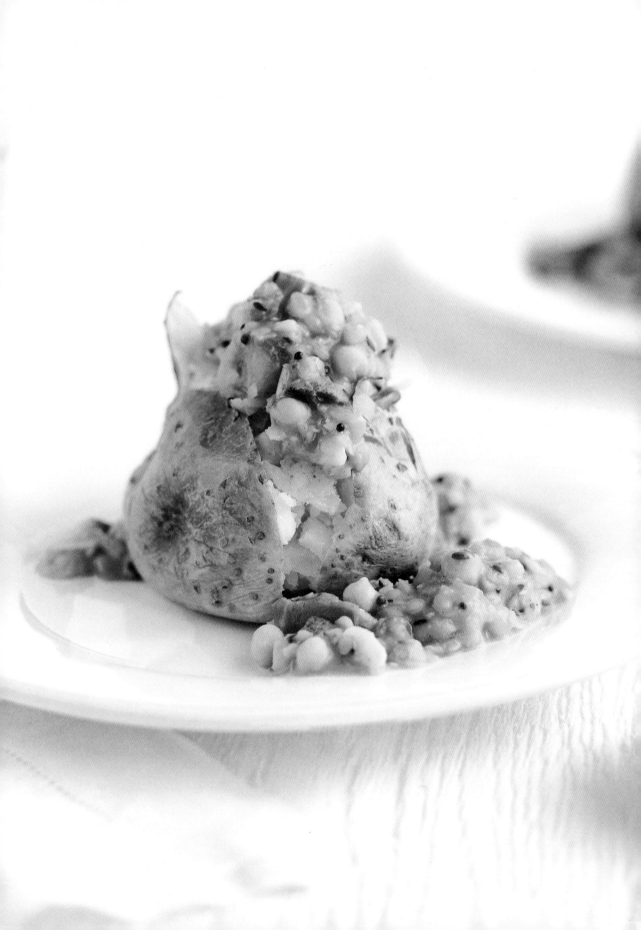

Sweet Potato & Lentil Soup

Lentils are a store cupboard essential – rich in protein and iron. Rinse well before use and add to stews, curries and soups like this comforting one.

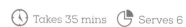 Takes 35 mins   Serves 6

- 2 tsp medium curry powder
- 3 tbsp olive oil
- 2 onions, grated
- 1 eating apple, peeled, cored and grated
- 3 garlic cloves, crushed
- 20g pack coriander, stalks chopped
- thumb-size piece fresh root ginger, grated
- 800g/1lb 12oz sweet potatoes
- 1.2 litres/2 pints vegetable bouillon
- 100g/4oz dried red lentils
- 300ml/½ pint milk
- juice 1 lime

1 Put the curry powder into a large saucepan, then toast over a medium heat for 2 mins. Add the olive oil, stirring as the spice sizzles in the pan. Tip in the onions, apple, garlic, coriander stalks and ginger, season, then gently cook for 5 mins, stirring every so often.

2 Meanwhile, peel, then grate the sweet potatoes. Tip into the pan with the stock, lentils, milk and seasoning, then simmer, covered, for 20 mins. Blend until smooth using a stick blender. Stir in the lime juice, check the seasoning and serve, topped with roughly chopped coriander leaves.

TIP Ginger contains potent anti-inflammatory compounds and helps settle an upset stomach.

BENEFITS low fat • vit C • fibre • 2 of 5 a day
PER SERVING 303 kcals • fat 8g • saturates 2g • carbs 44g • sugars 17g • fibre 7g • protein 9g • salt 0.71g

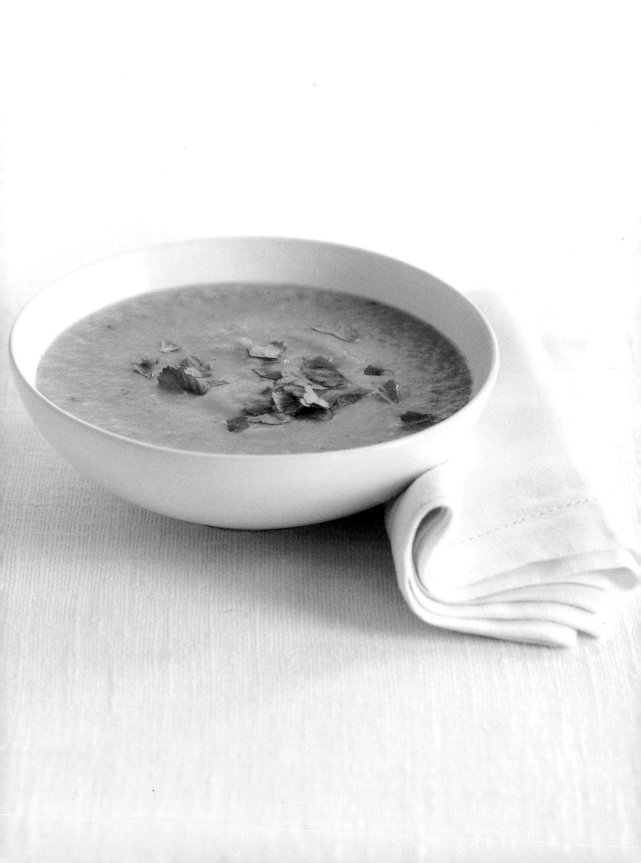

Asparagus Soup

If you have thin spears, no thicker than your little finger, then simply use the whole stalk. If the spears are the thickness of your thumb, then snap off the woody ends.

🕐 Takes 30 mins 🥧 Serves 4

- 25g/1oz butter
- a little rapeseed oil
- 350g/12oz asparagus spears, stalks chopped, woody ends discarded, tips reserved
- 3 shallots, finely sliced
- 2 garlic cloves, crushed
- 2 large handfuls spinach
- 700ml/1¼ pints vegetable bouillon
- olive oil, for drizzling (optional)

1 Heat the butter and oil in a large saucepan until foaming. Fry the asparagus tips for a few mins to soften. Remove and set aside.

2 Add the shallots, asparagus stalks and garlic, and cook for 5-10 mins until softened but still bright. Stir through the spinach, pour over the stock, bring to the boil, then blitz with a stick blender.

3 Season with black pepper and add hot water to loosen if needed. Ladle into bowls and scatter the asparagus tips over each. Drizzle with olive oil and serve.

BENEFITS vegetarian • low fat • folate • 1 of 5 a day
PER SERVING 101 kcals • fat 8g • saturates 4g • carbs 4g • sugars 4g • fibre 4g • protein 4g • salt 0.6g

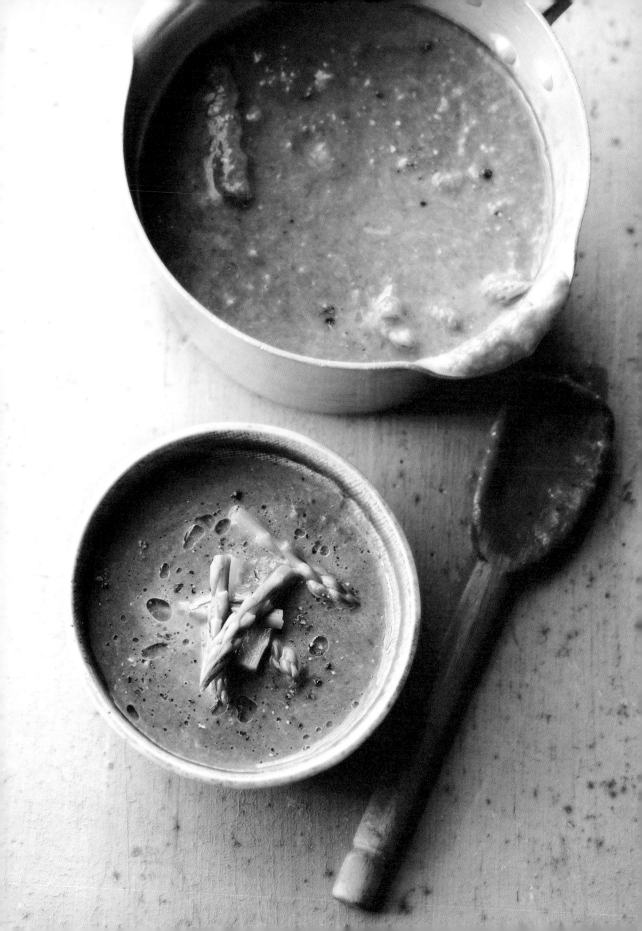

Veggie Wholewheat Pot Noodle

This clever packed lunch is super healthy, with crisp vegetables, wholewheat noodles and a spicy, zingy dressing.

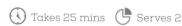 Takes 25 mins   Serves 2

- 100g/4oz dried wholewheat noodles
- 2 tsp rapeseed oil
- 1 red pepper, cut into fine strips
- ½ large courgette, cut into matchsticks
- 50g/2oz frozen shelled edamame beans
- 25g/1oz beansprouts
- 1 carrot, peeled and cut into matchsticks
- handful baby spinach
- 2 tbsp roughly chopped coriander

FOR THE DRESSING
- 1 tbsp sesame oil
- 2 tbsp lime juice
- 1 garlic clove, finely chopped
- 1 red chilli, deseeded and finely chopped
- 1 tsp grated ginger

1 Fill a large saucepan with water and bring to the boil. Add the noodles and cook for 3-5 mins or until tender. Drain and leave to cool.

2 Place a large non-stick pan (or wok) over a medium-high heat and add the oil. When hot, add the red pepper and cook for 2-3 mins until slightly softened. Add the courgette and edamame, and cook for a further 1-2 mins. Remove from the heat, transfer to a bowl and allow to cool.

3 Whisk together the dressing ingredients in a small bowl, or 2 jars if taking to work, then season.

4 Divide the noodles between 2 jars or plastic containers and top with the cooled vegetables, beansprouts, carrot, spinach and chopped coriander. Add the dressing just before eating.

BENEFITS vegan • low fat • 3 of 5 a day • fibre
PER SERVING 349 kcals • fat 11g • saturates 2g • carbs 47g • sugars 11g • fibre 9g • protein 12g • salt 1.0g

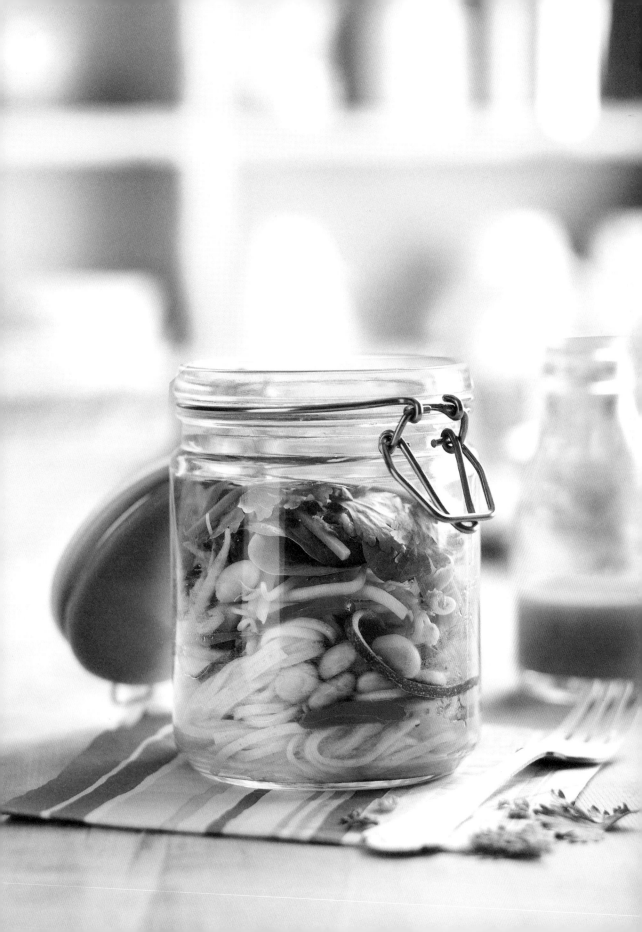

Lentil Ragu with Courgetti

This is a tasty meat-free Bolognese, delicious served on sweet potatoes, as well as these courgette noodles. Lentils are a rich plant source of energising iron as well as vitamin B1, which we need for a healthy nervous system. This makes quite a generous portion, but any leftovers will freeze well.

🕐 Takes 55 mins   🥧 Serves 4-6

- 2 tbsp rapeseed oil, plus 1 tsp
- 3 celery sticks, chopped
- 2 carrots, chopped
- 4 garlic cloves, chopped
- 2 onions, finely chopped
- 140g/6oz button mushrooms from a 280g pack, quartered
- 500g pack dried red lentils
- 500g pack passata
- 1 litre/1¾ pints reduced-salt vegetable bouillon
- 1 tsp dried oregano
- 2 tbsp balsamic vinegar
- 1-2 large courgettes, cut into noodles with a spiraliser, julienne peeler or knife

1 Heat the 2 tbsp oil in a large sauté pan. Add the celery, carrots, garlic and onions, and fry for 4-5 mins over a high heat to soften and start to colour. Add the mushrooms and fry for 2 mins more.

2 Stir in the lentils, passata, bouillon, oregano and balsamic vinegar. Cover the pan and leave to simmer for 30 mins until the lentils are tender and pulpy. Check occasionally and stir to make sure the mixture isn't sticking to the bottom of the pan; if it does, add a drop of water.

3 To serve, heat the remaining oil in a separate frying pan, add the courgette and stir-fry briefly to soften and warm through. Serve half the ragu with the courgetti and chill the rest to eat on another day. Can be frozen for up to 3 months.

TIP Cooking tomatoes or using them as a passata helps our bodies absorb more of their beneficial nutrient, lycopene. This helps lower cholesterol, strengthens blood vessels, boosts immunity and protects the eyes and skin.

BENEFITS vegetarian • low fat • folate • fibre • iron • 5 of 5 a day
PER SERVING (4) 578 kcals • fat 7g • saturates 1g • carbs 87g • sugars 19g • fibre 14g • protein 35g • salt 0.2g

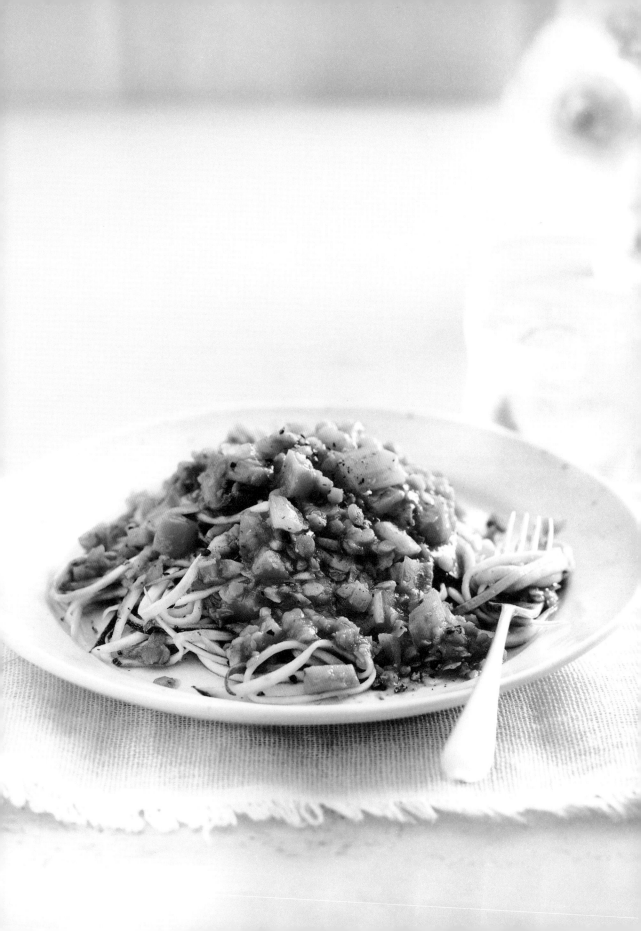

Moroccan Harira

This vegetarian version of the classic Moroccan soup contains turmeric, which is good for heart and brain health, and inflammatory conditions like arthritis. This makes enough for two meals and keeps well in the fridge.

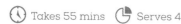 Takes 55 mins Serves 4

- 1-2 tbsp rapeseed oil
- 2 large onions, finely chopped
- 4 garlic cloves, chopped
- 2 tsp ground turmeric
- 2 tsp ground cumin
- ½ tsp ground cinnamon
- 2 red chillies, deseeded and sliced
- 500g carton passata
- 1.7 litres/3 pints reduced-salt vegetable bouillon
- 175g/6oz dried green lentils
- 2 carrots, chopped into pieces
- 1 sweet potato, peeled and diced
- 5 celery sticks, chopped into small pieces
- ⅔ small pack coriander, few sprigs reserved, the rest chopped
- 1 lemon, cut into 4 wedges, to serve

1 Heat the oil in a large non-stick sauté pan over a medium heat and fry the onions and garlic until starting to soften. Tip in the spices and chilli, stir briefly, then pour in the passata and stock. Add the lentils, carrots, sweet potato and celery, and bring to the boil.

2 Cover the pan and leave to simmer for 30 mins, then cook uncovered for a further 5-10 mins until the vegetables and lentils are tender. Stir in the chopped coriander and serve in bowls with lemon wedges for squeezing over, and the reserved coriander sprinkled over.

TIP Garlic is good for your skin as it is rich in sulphur, which helps to banish blemishes.

BENEFITS vegetarian • low fat • low cal • folate • fibre • vit c • iron • 4 of 5 a day
PER SERVING 335 kcals • fat 6g • saturates 1g • carbs 48g • sugars 21g • fibre 13g • protein 16g • salt 0.2g

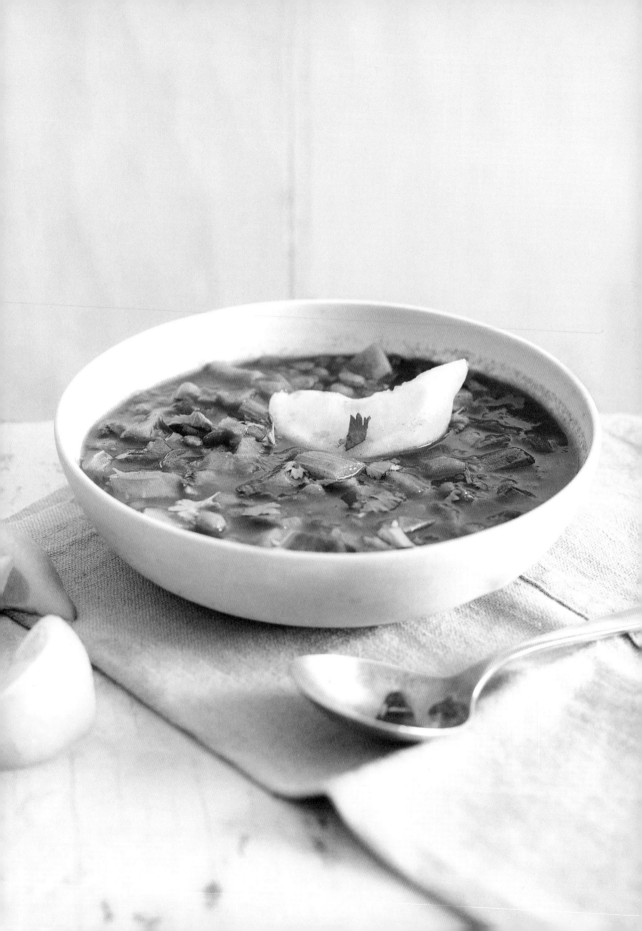

Barley & Broccoli Risotto with Lemon & Basil

This is packed with broccoli, which is a great anti-ager as it stimulates the energy-producers in our cells, making them more efficient. Barley lowers cholesterol, aids digestion and releases its energy slowly, helping to regulate appetite.

 Takes 45 mins, plus overnight soaking   Serves 2

- 100g/4oz wholegrain pearl barley
- 2 tsp reduced-salt vegetable bouillon powder
- 2 tbsp rapeseed oil
- 1 large leek, chopped
- 2 garlic cloves
- ⅔ pack basil
- generous squeeze of lemon juice
- 125g/4½oz Tenderstem broccoli from a 200g pack

1 Pour 1 litre/1¾ pints of cold water over the barley, cover and leave to soak overnight. Soaking the barley makes it quicker to cook and more digestible.

2 The next day, drain the barley, reserve the liquid and use it to make 500ml/18fl oz vegetable bouillon. Heat half the oil in a non-stick pan, add the leek and cook briefly to soften. Tip half into a bowl, then add the barley and bouillon to the pan, cover and simmer for 20 mins.

3 Meanwhile, add the garlic, basil, remaining oil, the lemon juice and 3 tbsp water to the leeks in the bowl, and blitz to a paste with a stick blender.

4 When the barley has cooked for 20 mins, add the broccoli to the pan and cook for 5-10 mins more until both are tender. Stir in the basil purée, heat very briefly (to retain the fragrance), then spoon into bowls to serve.

BENEFITS vegetarian • low cal • folate • fibre • vit c • iron • 2 of 5 a day
PER SERVING 378 kcals • fat 14g • saturates 1g • carbs 49g • sugars 5g • fibre 7g • protein 11g • salt 0.1g

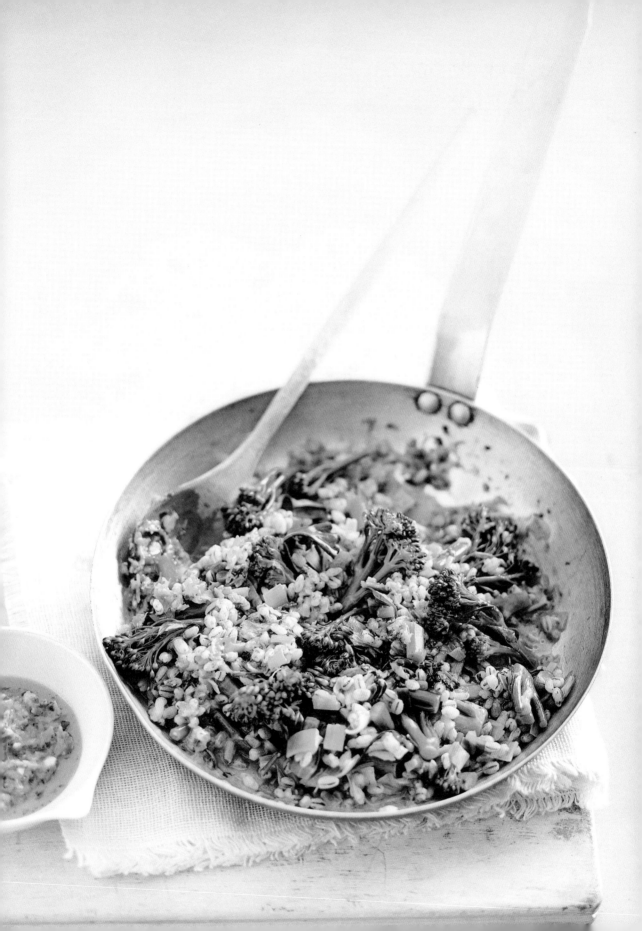

Sweet Potato Jackets
with Guacamole & Kidney Beans

Unlike regular potatoes, sweet potatoes count as 1 of your 5 a day. They also contain beta-carotene, a protective antioxidant. Although naturally sweet-tasting, they don't disrupt blood sugar levels.

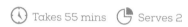 Takes 55 mins   Serves 2

- a drop of rapeseed oil
- 2 sweet potatoes
- 1 large avocado
- juice 1 lime, plus 2 wedges
- 1 red chilli, deseeded and finely chopped
- 2 tomatoes, finely chopped
- ⅓ small pack coriander, leaves roughly chopped
- 1 small red onion, finely chopped
- 400g can red kidney beans, drained

1 Heat oven to 220C/200C fan/gas 7. Oil the sweet potatoes, then put them straight on the oven shelf and roast for 45 mins or until tender all the way through when pierced with a knife.
2 Meanwhile, mash the avocado with the lime juice in a small bowl, then stir in the chilli, tomatoes, coriander and onion.
3 Cut the sweet potatoes in half and top with the beans and guacamole. Serve with the lime wedges for squeezing over.

TIP Kidney beans supply both soluble and insoluble fibre, and promote bowel regularity, essential for wellbeing.

BENEFITS vegan · folate · fibre · vit c · iron · 4 of 5 a day · gluten free
PER SERVING 586 kcals · fat 21g · saturates 4g · carbs 73g · sugars 31g · fibre 24g · protein 14g · salt 0.3g

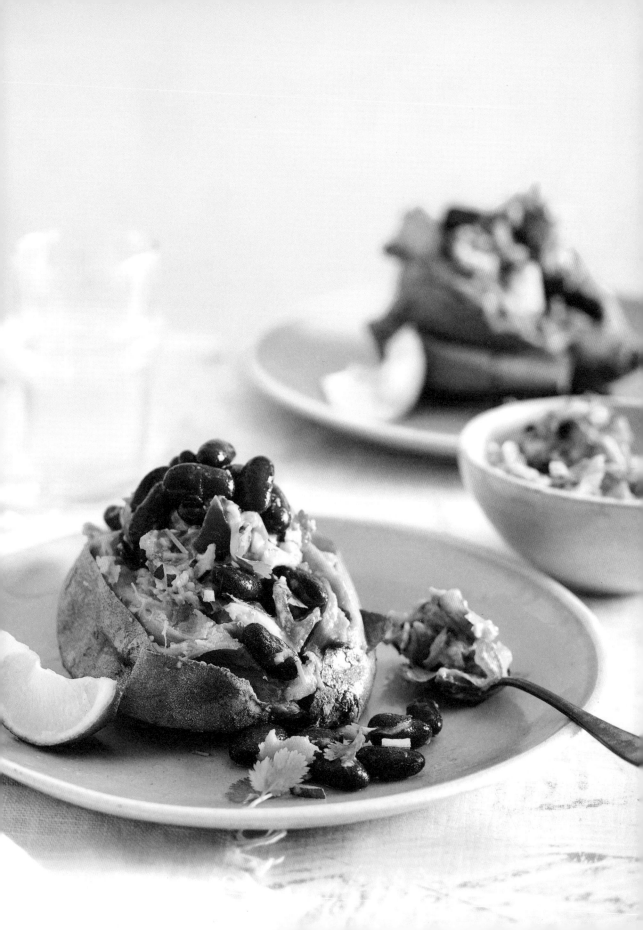

Niçoise Egg Salad

This makes a lovely lunch that is filling and full of flavour. Eggs are a useful protein for vegetarians and promote better short-term memory as well as being good for the skin and hair.

 Takes 20 mins   Serves 2

FOR THE SALAD
- 2 eggs
- 250g/9oz new potatoes, thickly sliced
- 200g/8oz fine green beans
- ½ red onion, very finely chopped
- 14 cherry tomatoes, halved
- 6 romaine lettuce leaves, torn into bite-sized pieces
- 6 pitted Kalamata olives, rinsed and halved

FOR THE DRESSING
- 2 tbsp rapeseed oil
- juice 1 lemon
- 1 tsp balsamic vinegar
- 1 garlic clove, grated
- ⅓ small pack basil, leaves chopped
- 3 pitted kalamata olives, rinsed and chopped

1 Boil the eggs for 8 mins in a small pan, making sure they are completely covered with water. Drain and cool in cold water then shell and halve. At the same time, boil the potatoes for 7 mins, add the beans and boil for 5 mins more or until both are just tender, then drain.

2 Mix the dressing ingredients together in a large bowl with 1 tbsp water. Toss the beans and potatoes with the other salad ingredients in half the dressing. Pile the salad on to plates, then top with the eggs and drizzle over the remaining dressing.

BENEFITS *low cal • folate • fibre • vit c • iron • 3 of 5 a day • gluten free*
PER SERVING *383 kcals • fat 20g • saturates 3g • carbs 31g • sugars 11g • fibre 12g • protein 14g • salt 0.7 g*

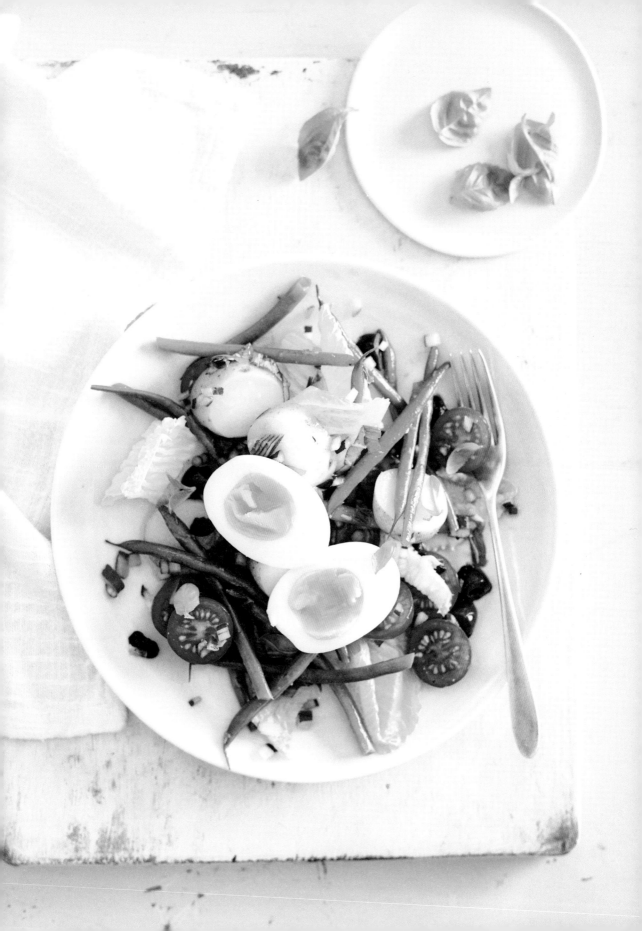

End-of-the-week Noodles with Ginger & Tamari

Make Friday night easy with this healthy, quick, yet filling supper. Nutrient-dense wholewheat noodles help keep blood sugar levels steadier than other carbs.

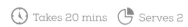 Takes 20 mins   Serves 2

- 1 nest wholewheat noodles (about 75g/3oz)
- 1 tbsp rapeseed oil
- 1 onion, halved and sliced
- 1 tbsp shredded ginger
- 2 garlic cloves, chopped
- about 115g/4oz button mushrooms, quartered
- about 65g/2½oz Tenderstem broccoli, chopped
- 50g/2oz mixed nuts, roughly chopped
- 2 carrots, cut into noodles with a spiralizer or julienne peeler
- 1 tbsp tamari
- ⅓ small pack coriander, roughly chopped

1 Pour boiling water over the noodles, leave them to soak for 5 mins, then drain.
2 Meanwhile, heat the oil in a wok and stir-fry the onion, ginger, garlic and mushrooms for 3-4 mins until starting to colour. Add the broccoli and nuts, and cook for a few mins more. Toss in the carrots and tamari, stir-fry until they just start to soften, then add the noodles and coriander.

TIP Fermented soya products such as tamari contain a type of carbohydrate that acts as fuel for friendly gut bacteria

BENEFITS vegan • low cal • folate • fibre • 3 of 5 a day
PER SERVING 430 kcals • fat 20g • saturates 2g • carbs 44g • sugars 14g • fibre 10g • protein 14g • salt 1.5g

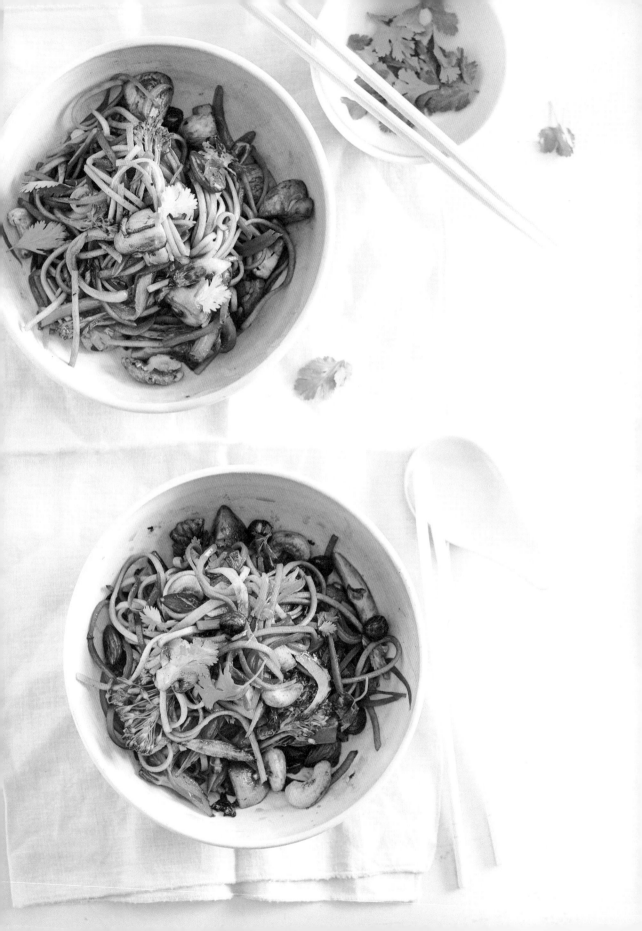

Toasted Sweetcorn, Avocado & Quinoa Salad

Try this vegan salad with protective carotenoids. Protein-packed quinoa is a popular gluten-free choice – it's loaded with stress-reducing magnesium as well as energizing B vitamins.

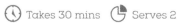 Takes 30 mins   Serves 2

- 75g/3oz quinoa
- 140g/5oz frozen sweetcorn
- 1 tbsp extra virgin olive or rapeseed oil
- 75g/3oz cherry tomatoes, quartered
- 1 small pack coriander, roughly chopped
- 2 spring onions, thinly sliced
- finely grated zest and juice 1 lime
- ½ long red chilli, finely chopped (deseeded if you don't like it too hot)
- 1 ripe avocado
- 25g/1oz mixed nuts, such as Brazils, almonds, hazelnuts, pecans and walnuts

1. Half fill a medium pan with water and bring to the boil. Rinse the quinoa in a fine sieve, then add to the water, stir well and simmer for about 12 mins or until just tender.
2. While the quinoa is cooking, put the sweetcorn in a dry frying pan and place over a medium-high heat. Cook for 5-6 mins, turning every now and then until lightly toasted. Set aside.
3. Rinse the cooked quinoa in a sieve under cold water, then press hard with a ladle or serving spoon to remove as much of the excess water as possible.
4. Tip the quinoa into a bowl and toss with the olive oil, sweetcorn, tomatoes, coriander, spring onions, lime zest and chilli. Season well with black pepper.
5. Halve and stone the avocado. Scoop out the flesh with a large metal spoon and cut into slices. Toss with the lime juice. Add the avocado and nuts to the salad and toss gently together before serving.

BENEFITS vegan • fibre • iron • vit C • folate • 3 of 5 a day • gluten free
PER SERVING 481 kcals • fat 31g • saturates 5g • carbs 37g • sugars 6g • fibre 6g • protein 12g • salt 0.1g

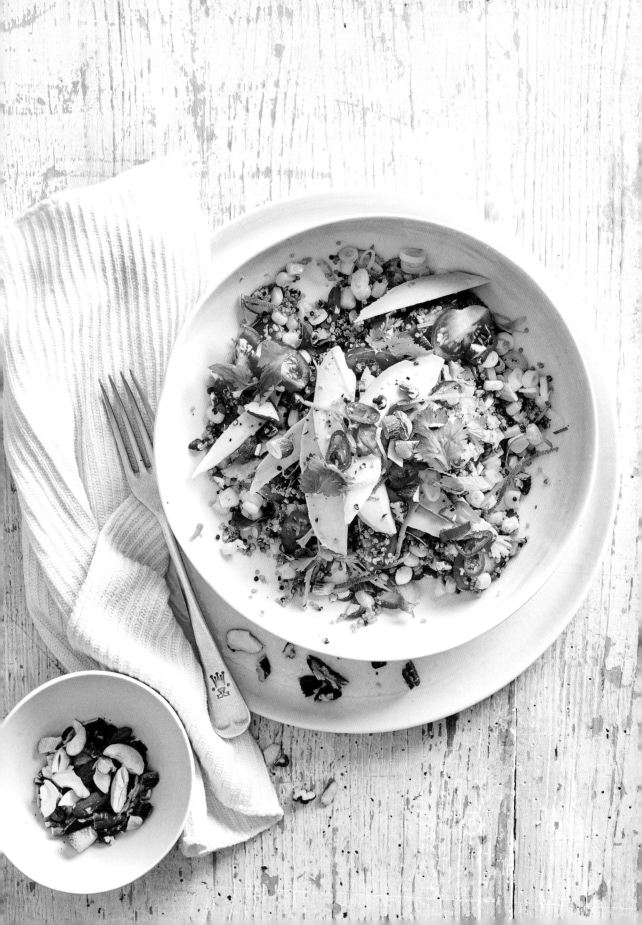

Roast Roots with Goat's Cheese & Spinach

This nutrient-dense supper is loaded with protective antioxidants from the broad range of vegetables as well as important immune-supportive minerals from our nut mix.

🕐 Takes 1 hour 25 mins   🥧 Serves 2

- 350g/12oz butternut squash, peeled and cut into chunks
- 200g/7oz carrots, peeled and cut into long batons
- 200g/7oz beetroot, scrubbed and cut into wedges
- 1 red onion, cut into wedges
- 1 tbsp rapeseed oil
- juice and finely grated zest 1 lemon
- 1 bulb garlic, cloves separated
- 4-5 thyme sprigs, roughly chopped
- 75g/3oz soft rindless goat's cheese log
- 25g/1oz mixed nuts, such as Brazils, almonds, hazelnuts, pecans and walnuts, roughly chopped
- 50g/2oz baby spinach

1 Heat oven to 200C/180C fan/gas 6. Put the vegetables, without the garlic, into a bowl and toss with the oil, lemon zest and juice and plenty of ground black pepper.

2 Scatter the vegetables over a large baking tray or roasting tin and bake for 30 mins. Take the tray out of the oven, add the garlic and thyme, then turn the vegetables. Return to the oven for 20 mins or until the vegetables are tender and lightly browned, turning halfway through.

3 Dot with the goat's cheese and nuts, scatter over the spinach and return to the oven for 3-5 mins or until the spinach has wilted and the goat's cheese has begun to melt. You can press the softened garlic cloves out of their skins and mash with the roasted vegetables, if you like.

BENEFITS *vegetarian • calcium • iron • fibre • vit C • folate • 5 of 5 a day • gluten free*
PER SERVING *561 kcals • fat 26g • saturates 8g • carbs 53g • sugars 33g • fibre 18g • protein 19g • salt 1g*

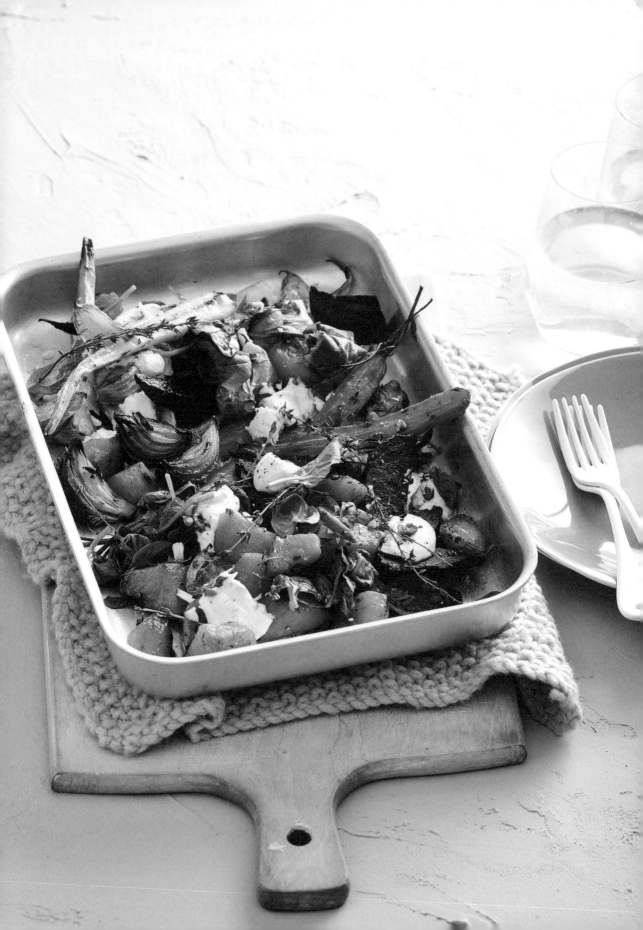

Chilli & Ginger Squash with Kale & Quinoa

This hearty 5 of your 5 a day supper easily serves two, with enough leftovers for lunch for one the next day

🕐 Takes 45 mins　◔ Serves 2

- 500g/1lb 2oz butternut squash, peeled and sliced
- 2 tbsp rapeseed oil
- ¼ tsp chilli flakes
- 1 onion, cut into wedges
- 1 red pepper, deseeded and thinly sliced
- 2 garlic cloves, very thinly sliced
- thumb-size piece of ginger, very thinly sliced
- 2 tsp each ground cumin and coriander
- 100g/4oz quinoa
- 100g/4oz green beans, trimmed and halved
- 100g/4oz frozen sweetcorn
- 75g/3oz shredded kale

1 Heat oven to 200C/180C fan/gas 6. Put the squash in a roasting tin and toss with 1 tbsp of the oil and lots of ground black pepper. Bake for 15 mins. Take out of the oven and turn the slices, sprinkle with the chilli flakes and return to the oven for a further 15-20 mins or until tender and lightly browned.

2 While the squash is roasting, heat the remaining oil in a large, wide-based non-stick saucepan pan or sauté pan. Add the onion and pepper to the pan and cook for 5 mins, stirring regularly until softened and lightly browned.

3 Add the garlic and ginger and stir-fry together for 1½ mins. Sprinkle over the cumin and coriander and fry for 30 secs, stirring. Stir in the quinoa, beans and sweetcorn. Pour over 600ml/1 pint just-boiled water, add ½ tsp flaked sea salt and bring to the boil, adding a splash more water if needed.

4 Reduce the heat to a simmer and cook for 12 mins, stirring regularly. Add the kale and continue cooking for a further 3 mins, or until the quinoa and vegetables are tender, stirring occasionally. Divide between 2 deep plates or bowls and top with the squash.

BENEFITS vegan • calcium • iron • vit C • folate • fibre • 5 of 5 a day • gluten free
PER SERVING 523 kcals • fat 16g• saturates 1g • carbs 72g • sugars 24g • fibre 11g • protein 17g • salt 1.2g

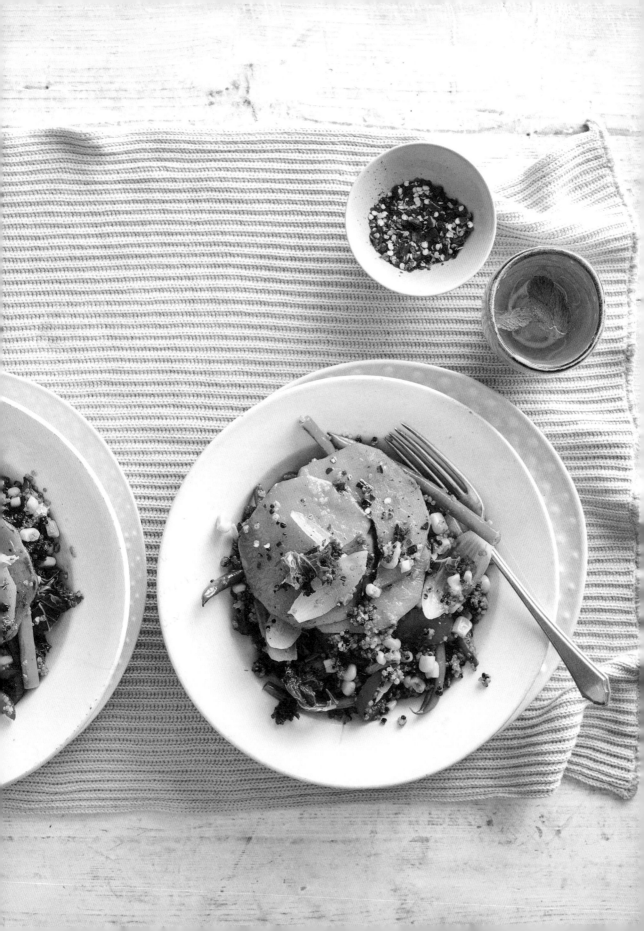

Chickpea & Nut Burgers with Sweet Potato Chips

These veggie burgers taste delicious hot or cold. Roll into small balls, making them into falafel if you prefer

 Takes 50 minutes 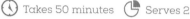 Serves 2

- 1 small red onion, roughly chopped
- 1 large garlic clove, halved
- 25g/1oz mixed nuts such as Brazils, almonds, hazelnuts, walnuts, pecans
- 1 tsp each ground cumin and coriander
- 400g can chickpeas, drained
- 25g/1oz wholemeal flour
- 1 small pack coriander
- 1 lemon, ½ juiced, plus ½ cut into wedges, to serve
- 2 tsp rapeseed oil

FOR THE CHIPS
- 300g/11oz sweet potatoes, cut into long wedges
- 1 tsp rapeseed oil

FOR THE SALAD
- 50g bag spinach and watercress salad
- 2 tomatoes, cut into wedges
- ⅓ cucumber, sliced
- 2 spring onions, thinly sliced
- 2 tsp balsamic vinegar

FOR THE YOGURT SAUCE
- 50g/2oz live bio yogurt
- 2 tbsp finely chopped mint

1 To make the yogurt sauce, stir together the yogurt and mint in a bowl and cover and chill until needed.
2 Heat oven to 220C/200C fan/gas 7. Half fill a medium saucepan with water and bring to the boil. Add the sweet potato wedges and cook for 4 mins then drain through a colander and return to the saucepan. Pour over the oil, tossing until lightly coated, then season with some ground black pepper.
3 Scatter the potatoes onto a small baking tray and roast for 15 mins. Take out of the oven and turn over, then cook for a further 10 mins or until tender and lightly browned.
4 While the chips are cooking, make the burgers. Put the onion, garlic, nuts and spices into a food processor and add lots of freshly ground black pepper. Blitz until as smooth as possible. Add the chickpeas, flour, coriander and lemon juice and blitz until the mixture comes together to make a thick paste. It shouldn't be too smooth as you are looking for some texture to give the burgers a bit of bite. Form the mixture into 4 balls and flatten into burgers, just under 2cm/¾in deep.
5 Heat 1 tsp of the oil in a medium non-stick pan over a low heat and cook the burgers on one side for 5 mins. Add the remaining 1 tsp of oil to the pan and turn over. Cook on the other side for a further 5 mins or until nicely browned and cooked throughout, keeping the heat low, so they don't burn.
6 Divide the salad leaves, tomatoes, cucumber and spring onions between 2 plates. Add the burgers, chips and mint sauce, plus a couple of lemon wedges for squeezing. Drizzle the balsamic vinegar over the salad and serve.

BENEFITS vegetarian • calcium • iron • vit C • fibre • 5 of 5 a day
PER SERVING 523 kcals • fat 19g • saturates 2g • carbs 63g • sugars 20g • fibre 14g • protein 19g • salt 0.4g

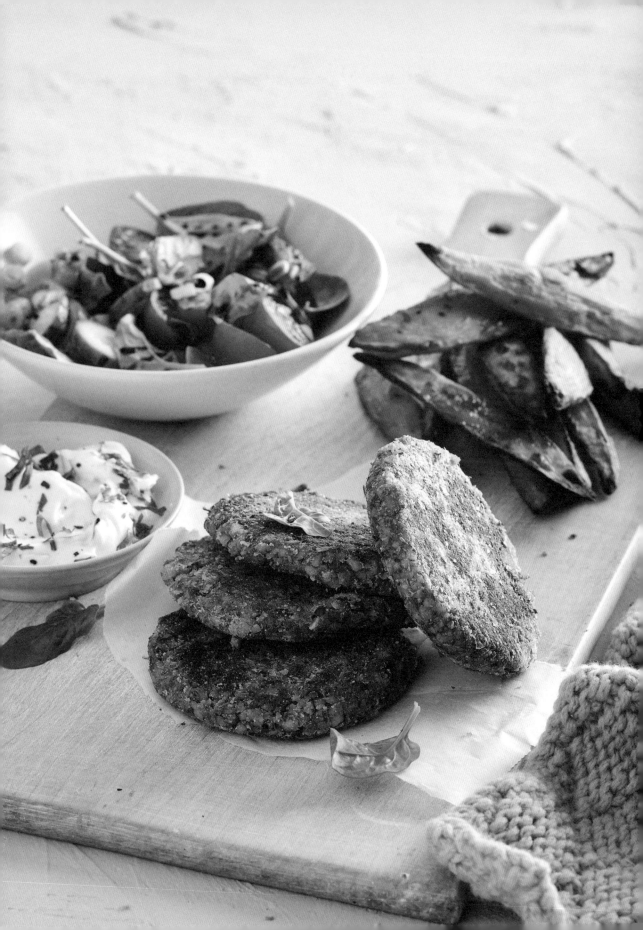

Moroccan Vegetable Stew

This warming one-pot stew is packed with nourishing ingredients like fibre-full chickpeas and iron-rich lentils

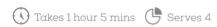 Takes 1 hour 5 mins Serves 4

- 1 tbsp rapeseed oil
- 1 onion, sliced
- 2 thin leeks, thickly siced
- 2 garlic cloves, sliced
- 2 tsp each ground cumin and coriander
- ½ tsp chilli flakes
- ¼ tsp ground cinnamon
- 400g chopped tomatoes
- 1 red and 1 yellow pepper, deseeded and cut into chunks
- 400g can chickpeas, drained
- 100g/4oz dried red lentils
- 375g/13oz sweet potatoes, peeled and cut into chunks
- juice 1 large orange, plus zest thickly sliced with a potato peeler
- 50g/2oz mixed nuts, such as Brazils, hazelnuts, pecans and walnuts, toasted and roughly chopped
- ½ small pack coriander, roughly chopped to serve
- live bio yogurt, to serve (optional)

1 Heat the oil in a large flameproof casserole or saucepan and gently fry the onion and leeks for 10-15 mins until well softened, stirring occasionally. Add the garlic and cook for 2 mins more.
2 Stir in the ground coriander, cumin, chilli and cinnamon. Cook for 2 mins, stirring occasionally. Season with plenty of ground black pepper. Add the chopped tomatoes, peppers, chickpeas, lentils, sweet potatoes, orange peel and juice, half the nuts and 400ml/14fl oz water and bring to a simmer. Cook for 15 mins, adding a splash of water if the stew looks too dry, and stir occasionally until the potatoes are softened but not breaking apart.
3 Remove the pan from the heat and ladle the stew into bowls. Scatter with coriander and the remaining nuts and top with yogurt, if using.

TIP Cumin improves blood circulation, while cinnamon is a digestive aid and helps regulate blood sugar levels.

*BENIFITS vegetarian • low cal • iron • vit C • folate • fibre • 5 of 5 a day • gluten free
PER SERVING 482 kcals • fat 14g • saturates 2g • carbs 63g • sugars 26g • fibre 15g • protein 18g • salt 0.6g*

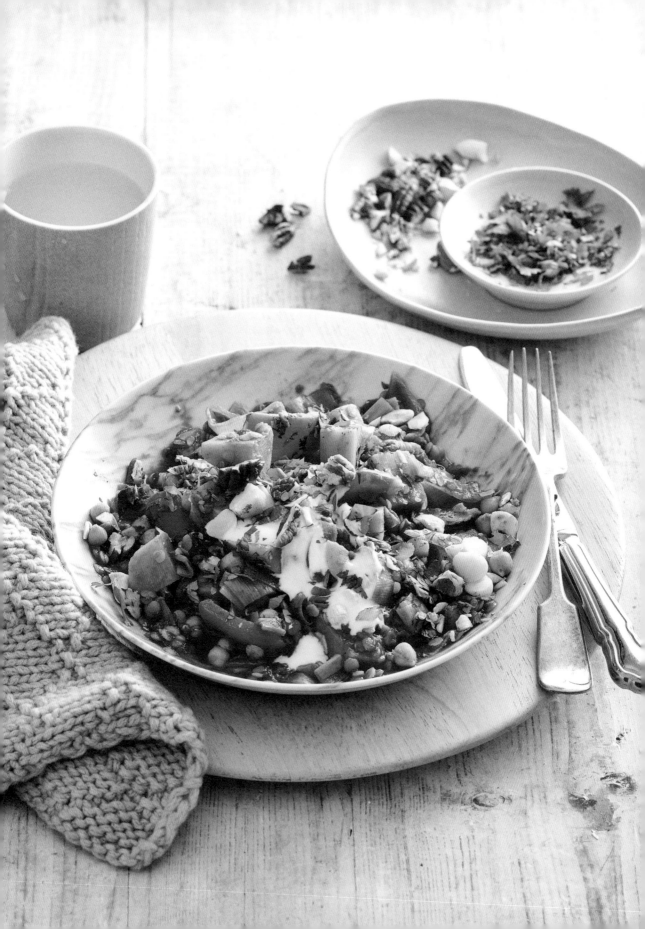

Miso-roasted Aubergine Steaks with Sweet Potato

Adding fabulous flavour to our aubergine steaks, miso is a valuable source of minerals, including iron as well as protein.

🕐 Takes 1 hour 25 mins   ◔ Serves 2

- 1 large aubergine (about 375g/13oz)
- 1½ tbsp brown miso paste (we used Clearspring)
- 350g/12oz sweet potatoes, unpeeled and cut into chunky wedges
- 1 tbsp rapeseed oil
- thumb-sized piece of ginger, grated
- 1 garlic clove, grated
- 8 spring onions, sliced diagonally
- small pack parsley, leaves chopped

1 Heat oven to 180C/160C fan/gas 4. Peel the aubergine with a potato peeler and roughly spread the miso paste all over it – the best way to do this is with the back of a spoon.

2 Put it in a roasting tin along with the sweet potato wedges. Pour 225ml/8fl oz boiling water into the base of the tin, then add the oil, ginger and garlic. Sprinkle a pinch of salt over the wedges and place in the oven.

3 After 30 mins, pour another 125ml/4½fl oz boiling water into the base of the tin and roast for another 20 mins. Repeat, adding 50ml/2fl oz boiling water and the spring onions, and roast for 10 mins more. Check the aubergine is cooked by inserting a knife in the centre – if it is ready it will easily slide in and out, and the aubergine will be soft on the inside.

4 Sprinkle the chopped parsley over the potato wedges, slice the aubergine into 2cm/¾in thick 'steaks' and serve on top of the potatoes. If there is no sauce in the bottom of the tin, add 3 tbsp water to loosen up the miso, then pour the miso gravy over the aubergine steaks and sprinkle with ground black pepper.

BENEFITS vegan • vit C • fibre • folate • low cal • 3 of 5 a day • gluten free • low fat
PER SERVING 341 kcals • fat 8g • saturates 1g • carbs 54g • sugars 30g • fibre 15g • protein 6g • salt 1.7g

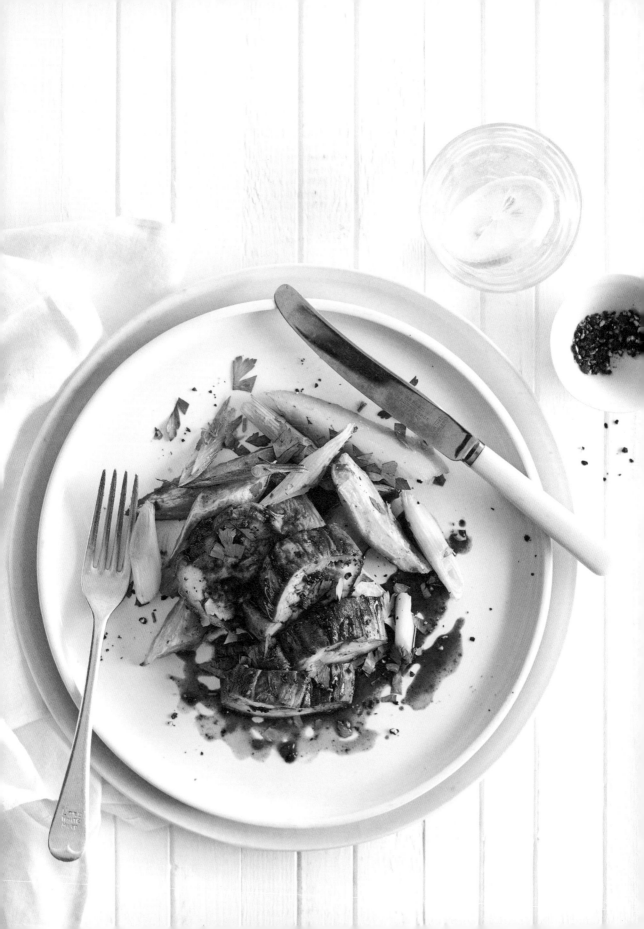

Sweet Potato Tex-Mex Salad

A hearty salad with lots of interesting flavours and textures.

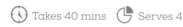 Takes 40 mins   Serves 4

- 600g/1lb 5oz sweet potatoes, cut into even chunks
- 2 tbsp extra virgin olive or rapeseed oil
- 1 tsp chilli flakes
- 400g can black beans, drained and rinsed
- 198g can sweetcorn, drained
- 2 avocados, chopped
- 250g/9oz tomatoes, cut into chunks
- 1 small red onion, thinly sliced
- 1 small pack coriander, roughly chopped
- juice 1 lime

1 Heat oven to 200C/180C fan/gas 6. On a baking tray, toss the sweet potato in 1 tbsp of the oil with the chilli flakes, sea salt and pepper. Roast for 30 mins until tender.
2 Once the sweet potato is nearly ready, combine the remaining ingredients in a large bowl with the remaining 1 tbsp oil and season well. Mix everything well but take care to avoid squashing the avocado. Divide the salad evenly among plates, or serve sharing-style, with the sweet potato chunks.

TIP Avocados supply more potassium than bananas. This, plus their rich monounsaturated fat content, makes them super healthy for the heart.

BENEFITS vegan • low cal • folate • fibre • vit c • 4 of 5 a day •gluten free
PER SERVING 485 kcals • fat 21g • saturates 4g • carbs 56g • sugars 27g • fibre 17g • protein 9g • salt 0.6g

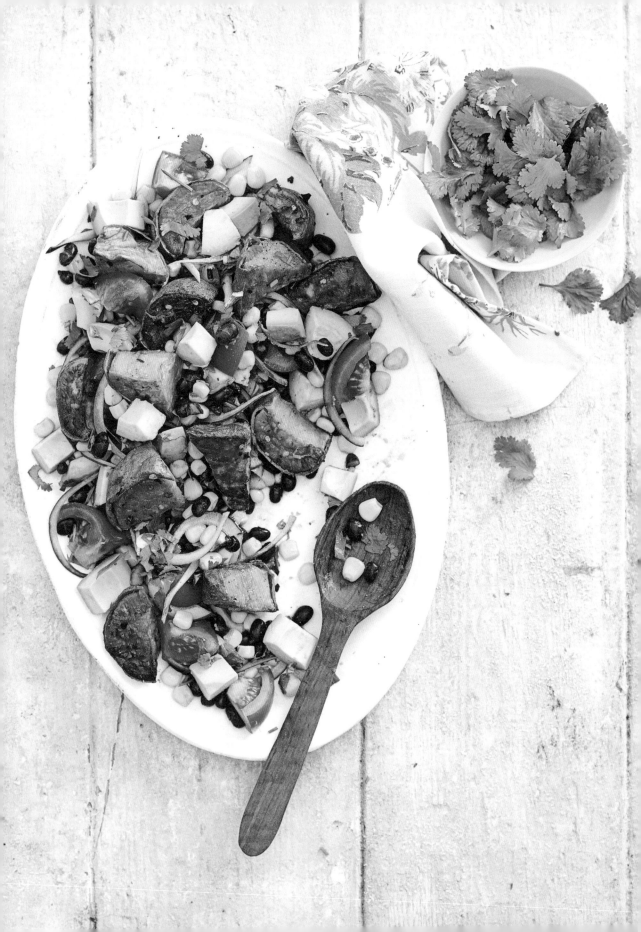

Radish, Lentil & Mint Salad

Here's a combo of sweet, sour and nutty ingredients to enhance the different varieties of beautiful radishes in this salad. Use a sharp, punchy apple cider vinegar, as the acidity will cut through the sweet onions and earthy lentils and bring the dish to life.

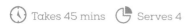 Takes 45 mins Serves 4

- 50g/2oz walnut pieces
- 3 tbsp olive oil
- 1 red onion, sliced
- 1 tsp black treacle
- 2 tbsp apple cider vinegar
- small pack mint, leaves picked and ½ chopped
- 400g can green lentils, drained and rinsed
- ½ cucumber, chopped
- 300g/11oz radishes, some left whole, others sliced and chopped (try to use a mixture of varieties, such as mooli and red meat radishes)

1 Toast the walnut pieces in a large frying pan over a medium heat until fragrant and just starting to char at the edges. Tip into a bowl and set aside.

2 In the same pan, turn the heat down to low and add 1 tbsp olive oil. Add the onion, fry gently for around 10 mins until soft, then take the pan off the heat. Add the black treacle, vinegar and the rest of the olive oil, then mix and leave to cool. Add the chopped mint to the pan, and season well.

3 In a large bowl, mix together the lentils, cucumber and half the radishes, then pour over the cooled onion and mint dressing. Toss everything together and pile into a serving dish. Scatter over the walnut pieces and the rest of the mint and radishes, then serve.

BENEFITS vegan • 3 of 5 a day • gluten free
PER SERVING 236 kcals • fat 17g • saturates 2g • carbs 11g • sugars 5g • fibre 4g • protein 6g • salt 0.1g

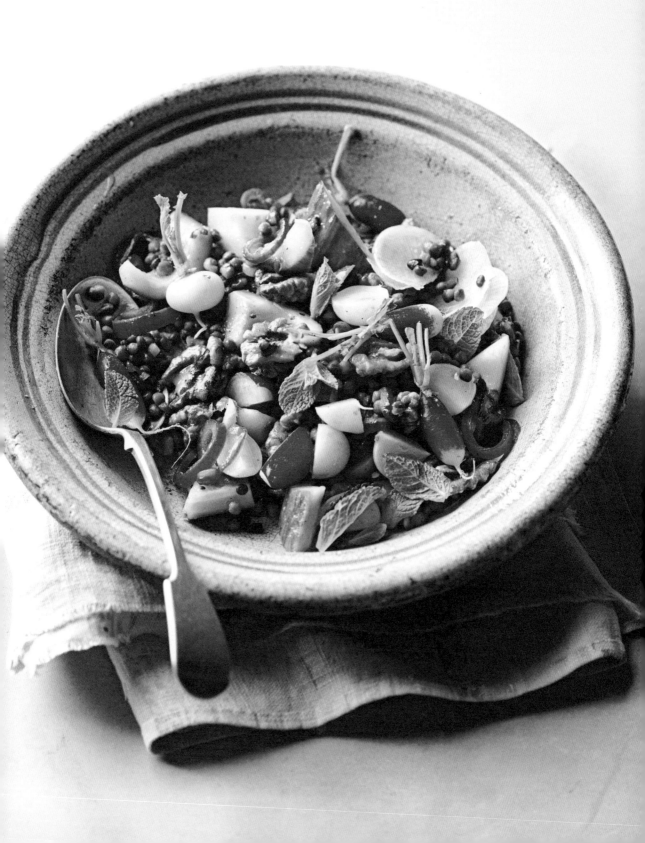

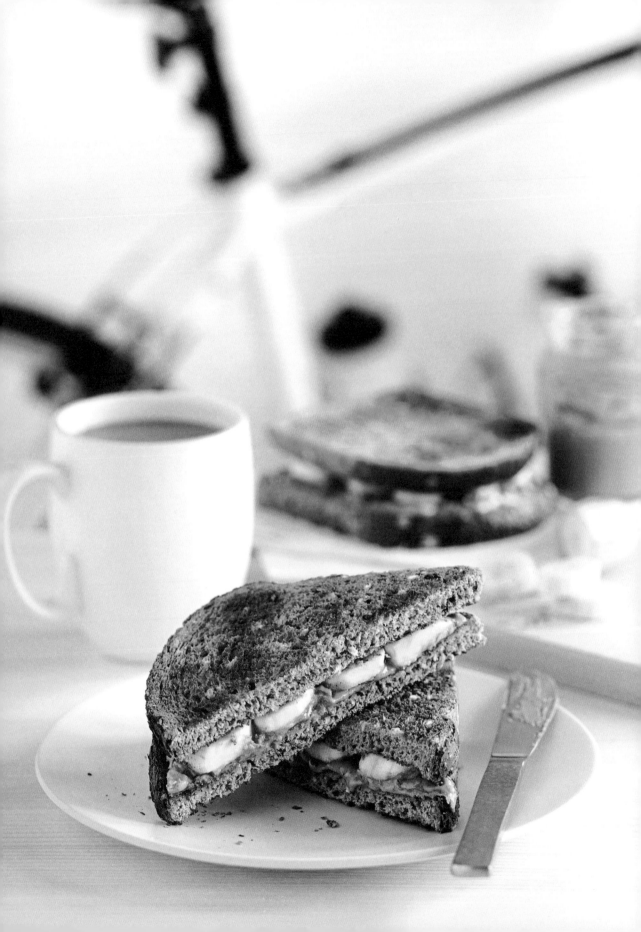

Chapter 4:

NUTRITIOUS SNACKS

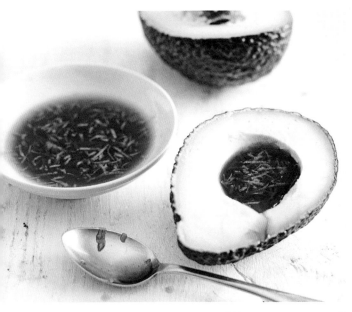

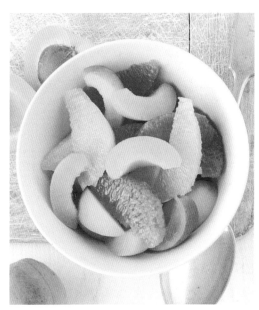

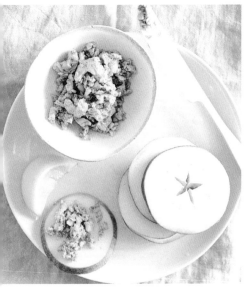

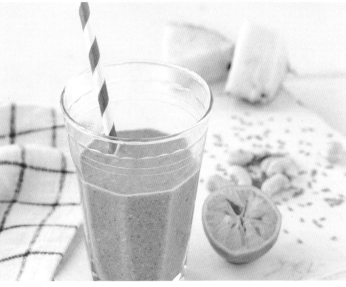

Snacks you can eat between meals

Our 7-day plans are designed to provide about 1500 calories a day, however, if you have a very active lifestyle or you feel you need to eat more regularly during the day this chapter includes a range of good for you snacks.

Snacking needn't mean a load more sugar and salt in your diet – our snacks are nutritious and filling yet full of flavour. The key to successful snacking is all about feeling satisfied. Fibre as well as protein and fats, all help to keep you full and happy. We've used ingredients like nut butter and tahini, which are high in 'good for you' fats as well as protein. In fact, peanut butter contains as much as 4g of protein in each tablespoon so it's ideal for satisfying cravings – even sweet ones. Along with these ingredients, we've used beans, whole-grains and fruit like apples, which are rich sources of fibre.

Snack time is the perfect opportunity to top up your 5 a day too, but don't just think of fruit. Our Edamame & chilli dip with crudités (page 232) is perfect for sneaking in some extra veggies and our Avocado with tamari & ginger dressing (page 244) makes a delicious, almost decadent, change from more traditional savoury snacks.

Snacking has its place in a healthy, balanced diet as long as you make the right choices and for the right reasons. Don't snack mindlessly or out of boredom – eat when you are hungry or when you know your next meal may be delayed. If time is short and you've not prepared a healthy snack, keep some simple, nutrient-dense foods to hand like unsalted nuts and seeds combined with a little dried fruit – a cupped handful will help tide you over to your next meal. Ideally don't snack after 8pm.

So go ahead, swap your regular snack for one or more of our nutritious nibbles and you'll not look back.

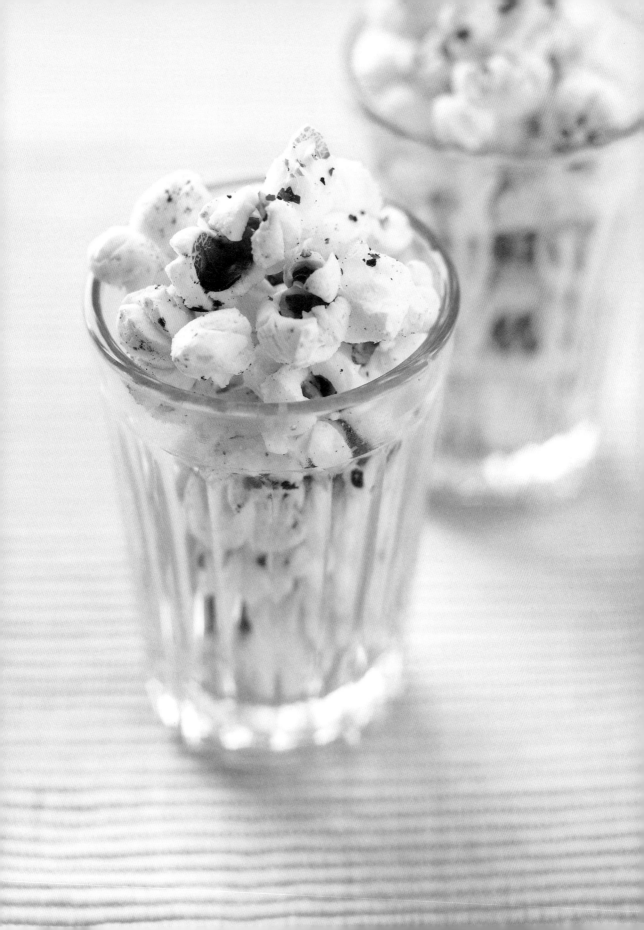

Smashed Bean Dip

Making your own houmous takes minutes to whizz together and creates a healthy starter to a meal, as well as a sustaining snack.

Takes 5 mins • Serves 3

- 400g can chickpeas, don't drain
- 400g can cannellini beans, drained
- zest and juice 1 lemon
- 2 garlic cloves, chopped
- 2 tsp ground cumin
- 100ml/3fl oz live bio yogurt
- vegetable sticks for dipping, to serve
- pine nuts and sunflower and pumpkin seeds for sprinkling, optional

1 Tip the chickpeas into a sieve set over a bowl or jug to catch the liquid. Tip the chickpeas and beans into a food processor or blender with the lemon juice and zest, garlic, cumin and yogurt, and whizz to a rough paste.
2 Whizz in a tbsp of the chickpea liquid at a time if necessary until you have a dipping consistency, then scrape into a bowl. Serve with veg sticks and a sprinkling of the nuts and seeds if you like. This will keep in the fridge for a couple of days.

BENEFITS vegetarian • 1 of 5 a day • gluten free
PER SERVING 172 kcals • fat 5g • saturates 1g • carbs 22g • sugars 3g • fibre 3g • protein 11g • salt 1.04g

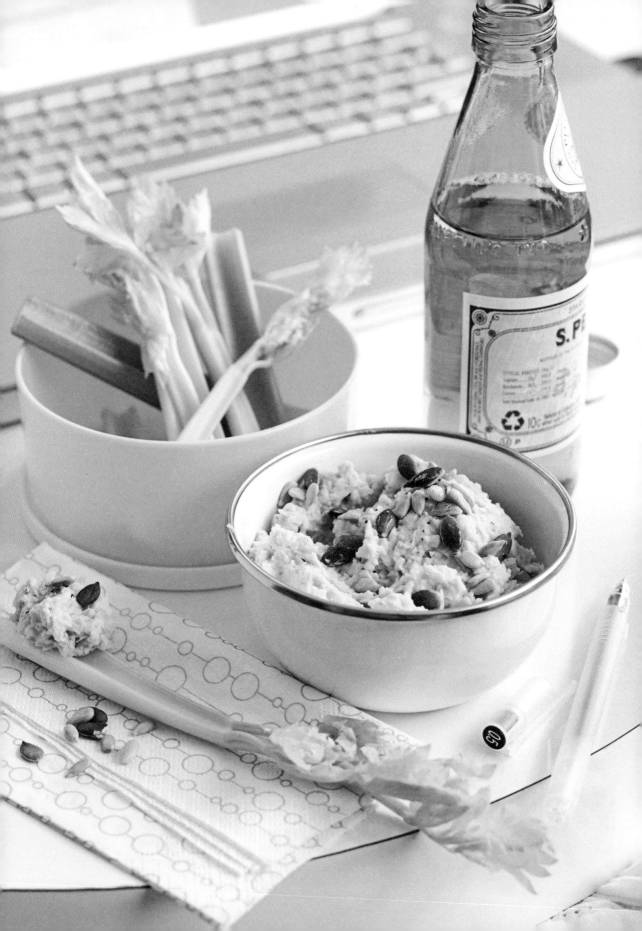

Edamame & Chilli Dip

This is easily halved if you don't want to make eight portions, but it will keep in the fridge or freeze. Up the veggie servings by allowing half a pepper, a carrot and celery stick with a generous serving of radishes for dipping per person. Soya beans are a great high protein, low fat choice.

🕐 Takes 15 mins   🥧 Serves 8

- 300g/11oz frozen soya beans (edamame)
- 150g pot live bio yogurt,
- 1 chopped red chilli (deseeded if you don't like it too hot)
- juice 1 lime
- 1 garlic clove, crushed
- 1 red onion, finely chopped
- handful chopped coriander
- halved radishes and sticks of carrots, celery and peppers, to serve

1 Cook the beans in boiling water for 4 mins. Drain and cool under cold running water. Tip into a food processor and blitz with the yogurt, chilli, lime juice and garlic until smooth.

2 Stir in the finely chopped red onion and coriander. Serve with halved radishes and sticks of carrots, celery and peppers. The dip will keep covered in the fridge for up to 3 days.

BENEFITS vegetarian • low fat • gluten free
PER SERVING 71 kcals • fat 3g • saturates 1g • carbs 6g • sugars 2g • fibre 2g • protein 6g • salt 0.4g

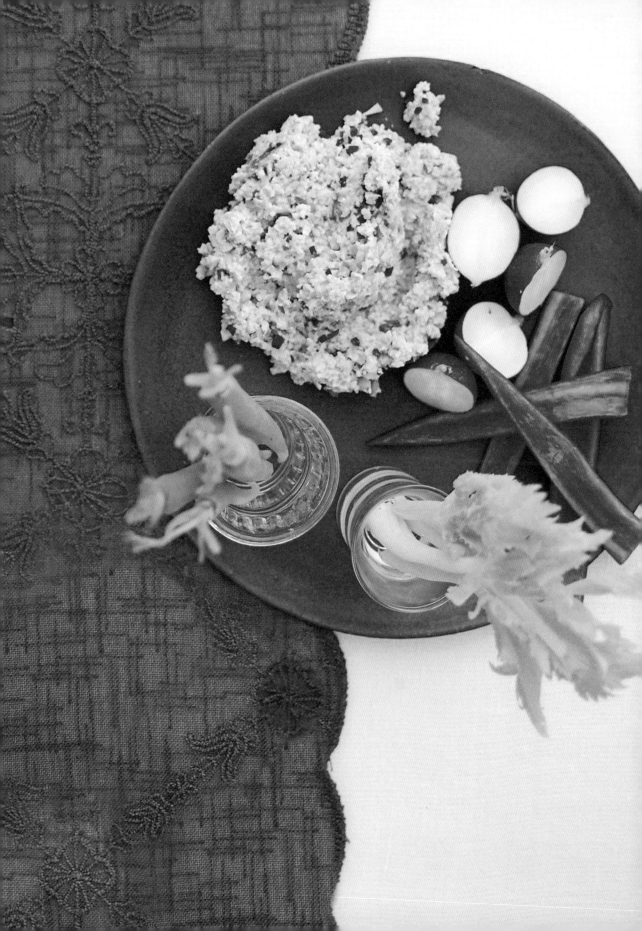

Spicy Roast Chickpeas

Chickpeas are a useful source of iron for vegetarians and these savoury ones make a delicious change to peanuts or crisps.

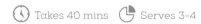 Takes 40 mins   Serves 3-4

- 400g can chickpeas, drained
- 1 tsp rapeseed oil
- 1 tsp each smoked paprika, cumin and coriander

1 Heat oven to 180C/160C fan/gas 4. Tip the chickpeas into a bowl and toss with the rapeseed oil, smoked paprika, cumin and coriander.

2 Toss well until the chickpeas are well coated in the spices, then tip out onto a baking tray and bake for 35 mins, moving them round the tray halfway through so they dry out evenly and are crunchy. Leave to cool, then store in an airtight container. They will keep for a few days.

BENEFITS vegan • 1 of 5 a day • gluten free
PER SERVING (3) 115 kcals • fat 3g • saturates 0.3g • carbs 12g • sugars 0.4g • fibre 5g • protein 6g • salt 0g

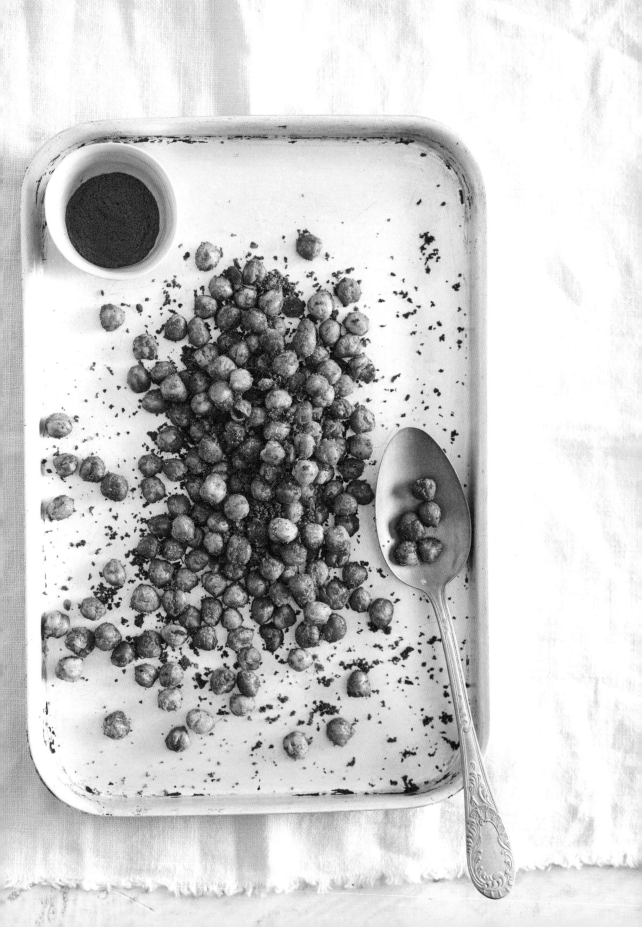

Chilli Popcorn

A guilt-free treat that is sure to fill you up.

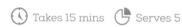 Takes 15 mins   Serves 5

- 100g/4oz popcorn kernels
- 1 tsp chilli flakes
- 1 tsp freshly ground black pepper
- 2 tsp ground mixed spice

1 Heat oven to 200C/180C fan/gas 6. Pop the popcorn kernels according to the pack instructions.
2 Meanwhile, mix together the chilli flakes, freshly ground black pepper and mixed spice. Toss the popcorn with the spice mix, then tip on to a large baking sheet and put in the oven for 5 mins until the corn is crisp and the spices are fragrant.
3 Eat warm or once cooled. Will keep in an airtight container for up to a week.

BENEFITS vegan • gluten free
PER SERVING 128 kcals • fat 9g • saturates 1g • carbs 11g • sugars trace • fibre 0g • protein 2g • salt 0.02g

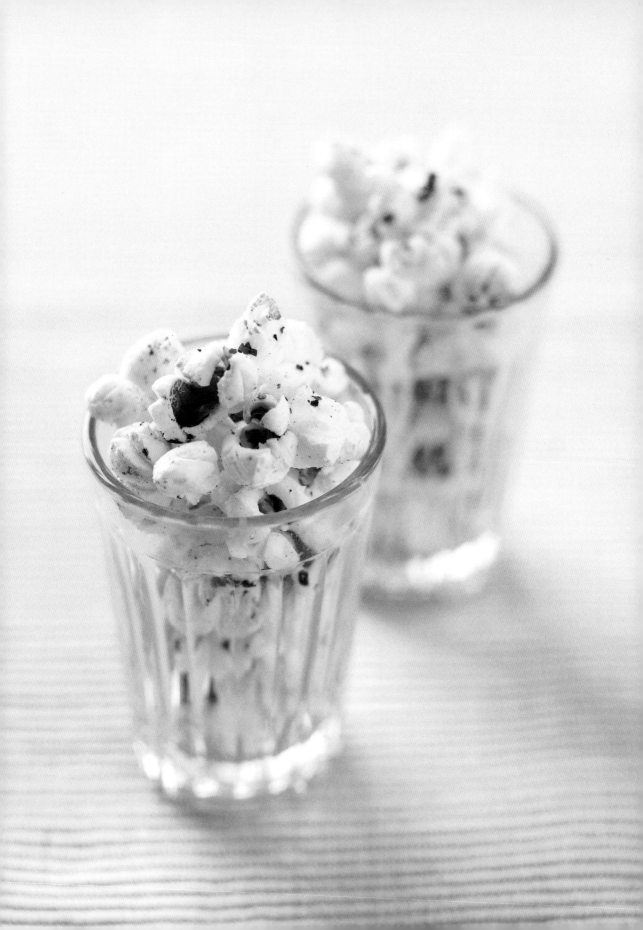

Cinnamon Cashew Spread with Apple Slices

Don't keep nut butters for toast and crackers – dollop a tablespoon into a homemade curry (just before serving) to add depth and creaminess.

🕐 Takes 10 mins   🥧 Makes 2

- 50g/2oz unroasted cashew nuts
- 1 tbsp coconut oil
- ½ tsp ground cinnamon
- 2 apples, sliced straight across into rounds
- 2 generous lemon wedges

1 Put the cashew nuts in a small bowl and pour over enough boiling water to cover them. Leave for 2-3 mins so they soften a little. Drain, and then return to the bowl.
2 Add the coconut oil and cinnamon and blitz with a stick blender to chop the nuts into a rough paste.
3 Serve with the apple slices and lemon wedges for squeezing over.

BENEFITS vegan • 1 of 5 a day •gluten free
PER SERVING 239 kcals • fat 18g • saturates 7g • carbs 12g • sugars 9g • fibre 3g • protein 6g • salt 0g

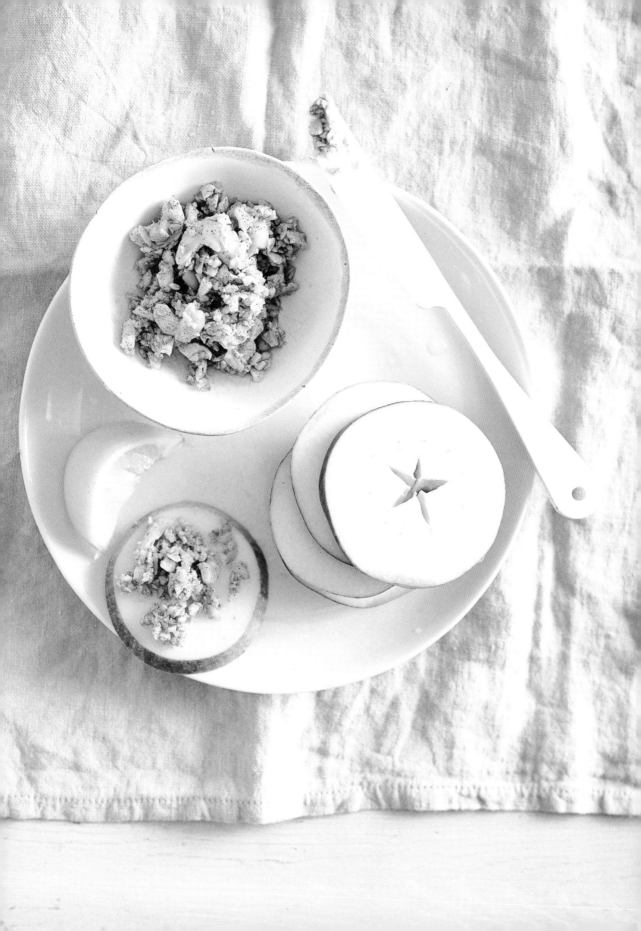

Almond Butter

Blitz up your own homemade nut butter for spreading on toast for a speedy snack or for adding to smoothies

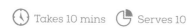 Takes 10 mins   Serves 10

- 250g/9oz blanched almonds
- 2 tbsp olive or coconut oil

1 Put the almonds in a food processor and blitz on high speed until finely chopped and the nuts have come together to form a thick ball. With the processor still running, add the oil, a little at a time, until the mixture is a smooth, glossy paste – about 7 mins.
2 Spoon into a clean jar, and keep tightly closed and refrigerated when not in use. Will keep in the fridge for up to 3 weeks.

BENEFITS vegan • gluten free
PER SERVING 158 kcals • fat 15g • saturates 1g • carbs 2g • sugars 1g • fibre 2g • protein 5g • salt 0g

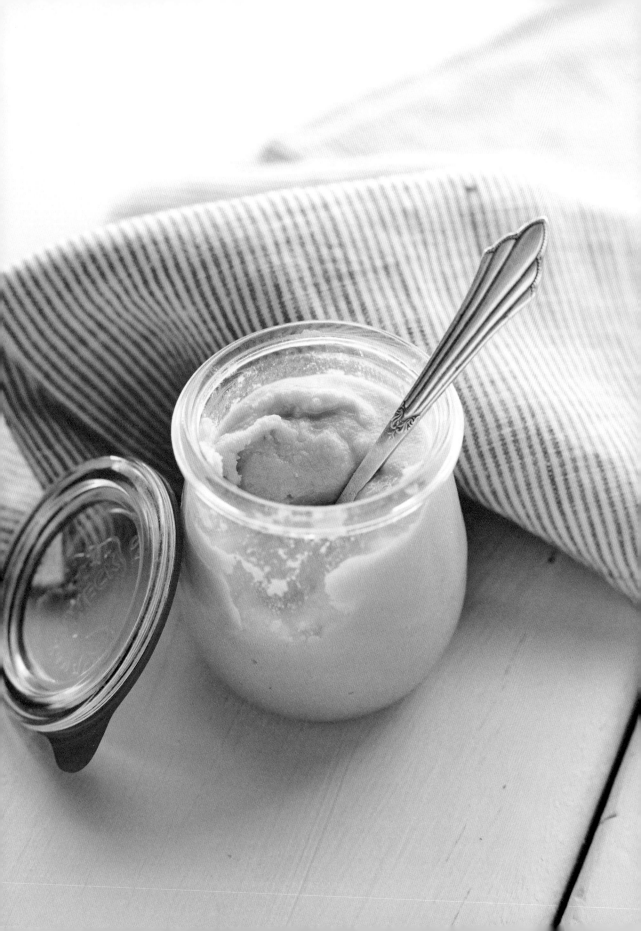

Peanut Butter & Banana on Toast

Here's a great snack for after exercise. Carbs help to refuel muscles by replenishing all-important glycogen stores. Eat it along with a glass of fruit juice or a milky drink.

🕙 Takes 10 mins   🕐 Serves 2

- 2 slices wholemeal or granary bread (see recipe for Seeded wholemeal loaf on page 268)
- 2 small bananas, sliced
- 1 tsp ground cinnamon
- 2 tbsp crunchy peanut butter

1 Toast the bread and layer the banana on one slice and dust with the cinnamon. Spread the second slice with the peanut butter, then sandwich them together and eat straight away.

BENEFITS vegetarian • folate • 1 of 5 a day
PER SERVING 307 kcals • fat 9g • saturates 2g • carbs 45g • sugars 18g • fibre 4g • protein 11g • salt 1.0g

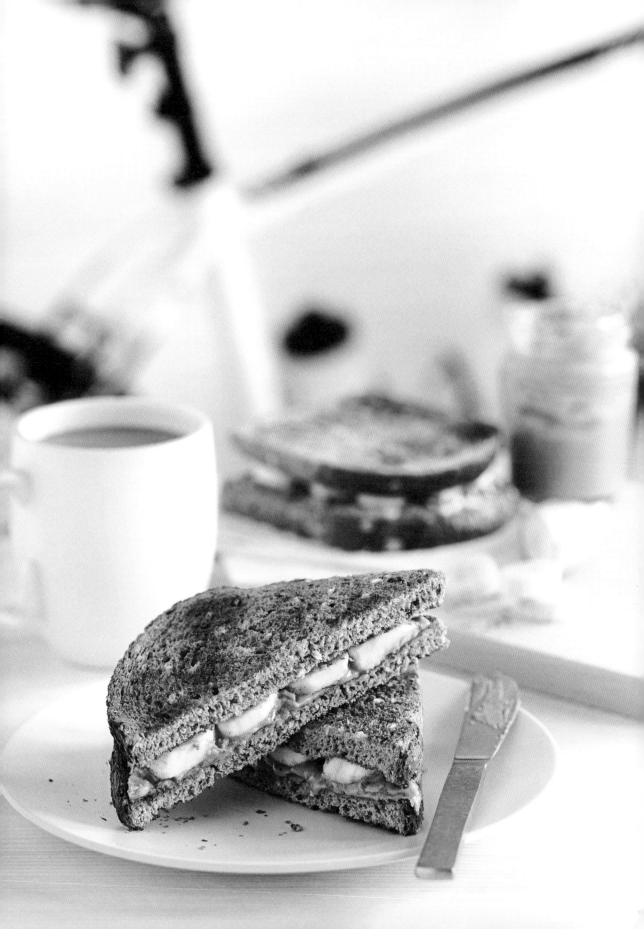

Avocado with Tamari & Ginger Dressing

Packed with skin-friendly vitamin E and anti-inflammatory ginger, this is a seriously good for you snack.

🕐 Takes 5 mins   ◑ Serves 2

- 1 small garlic clove, grated
- ½ tsp shredded ginger
- 1 tsp wheat-free tamari
- 2 tsp lemon juice
- 1 avocado, halved and stoned

1 Mix the garlic and ginger with the tamari and lemon juice in a small bowl, then dilute with 1-2 tsp water.

2 Spoon the dressing into the hollow of the avocado, where the stone came from, and eat with a teaspoon.

BENEFITS vegan • 1 of 5 a day • gluten free
PER SERVING 148 kcals • fat 14g • saturates 3g • carbs 2g • sugars 1g • fibre 3g • protein 2g • salt 0.4g

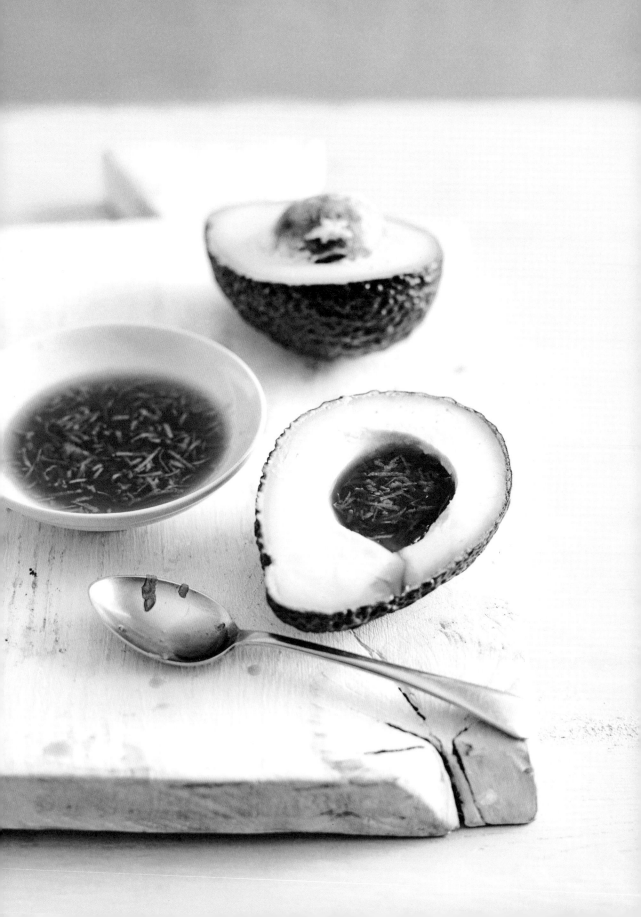

Curried Turkey Lettuce Wraps

Ditch the bread for these lettuce wraps – they're a clever balance of protein and carbs.

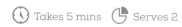 Takes 5 mins Serves 2

- 100g/4oz live bio yogurt
- 1 tsp curry powder
- 1 tsp tomato purée
- 2 tbsp raisins
- 100g/4oz cooked skinless turkey or chicken breast meat, chopped
- 8 Little Gem lettuce leaves
- 2 tsp sunflower seeds
- few coriander leaves

1 Mix the yogurt with the curry powder, tomato purée and raisins. Stir in the turkey or chicken, then spoon onto the Little Gem lettuce leaves. Scatter over the sunflower seeds and coriander leaves and serve.

BENEFITS low fat • 1 of 5 a day
PER SERVING 235 kcals • fat 5g • saturates 2g • carbs 25g • sugars 24g • fibre 2g • protein 22g • salt 0.2 g

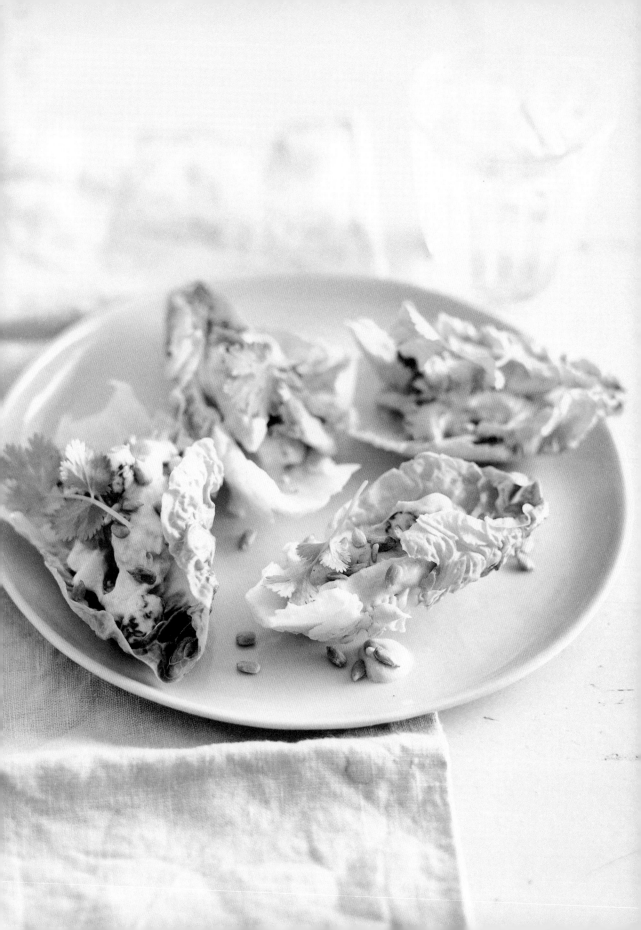

Energy Bites

Instead of reaching for the biscuit tin, shape a mix of nut butter, flaxseeds, pecans, raisins and coconut into balls for a healthy, energy-boosting treat that is just as tasty.

🕐 Takes 10 mins, plus 20 mins chilling   🥧 Serves 8

- 100g/4oz pecans
- 75g/3oz raisins
- 2 tbsp peanut or Almond butter (page 240)
- 1 tbsp ground flaxseeds (or a mix such as milled flaxseed, almonds, Brazil nuts and walnuts)
- 1 tbsp cocoa
- 1 tbsp maple syrup
- 50g/2oz desiccated coconut

1 Put pecans in a food processor and blitz to crumbs. Add raisins, nut butter, flaxseeds, cocoa and syrup, then pulse to combine.
2 Shape the mixture into golf ball-sized balls and roll in the desiccated coconut to coat. Put in the fridge to firm for 20 mins.

BENEFITS vegan • gluten free
PER BITE 204 kcals • fat 17g • saturates 5g • carbs 10g • sugars 10g • fibre 3g • protein 4g • salt 0.1g

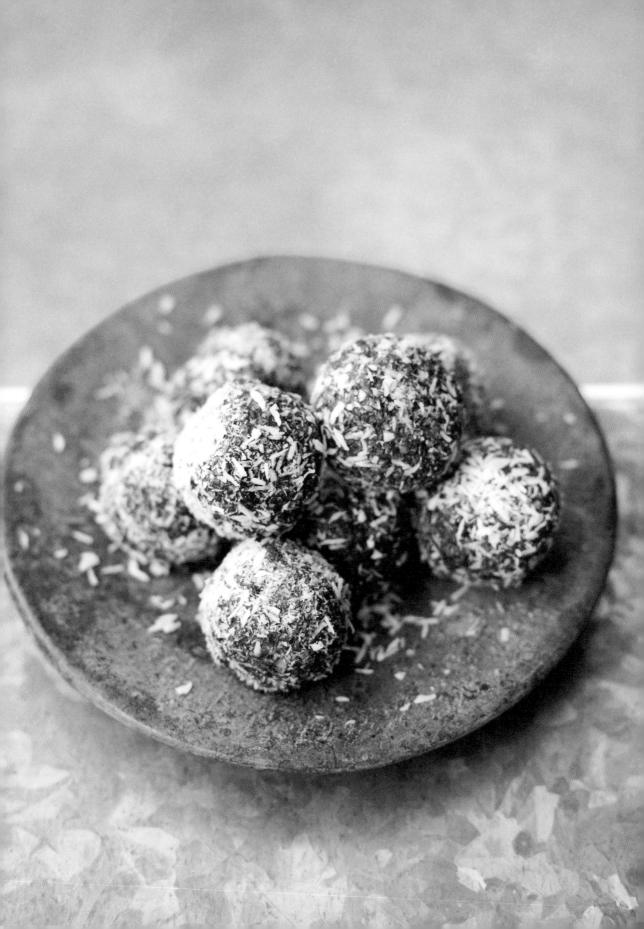

Berry Omelette Pancake

This high-protein snack is a one-egg omelette cleverly disguised as a pancake. When berries are not in season, try chopped banana with a sprinkle of cinnamon.

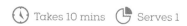 Takes 10 mins   Serves 1

- 1 large egg
- 1 tbsp milk or water
- 3 pinches of ground cinnamon
- ½ tsp rapeseed oil
- 100g/4oz cottage cheese
- 175g/6oz chopped strawberries, blueberries and raspberries

1 Beat the egg with the milk or water and cinnamon. Heat the oil in a 20cm/8in non-stick frying pan and pour in the egg mixture, swirling to evenly cover the base. Cook for a few mins until set and golden underneath. There's no need to flip it over.
2 Place on a plate, spread over the cheese, then scatter with the berries. Roll up and serve.

BENEFITS vegetarian • folate • vit C • 2 of 5 a day • gluten free
PER SERVING 264 kcals • fat 12g • saturates 4g • carbs 18g • sugars 16g • fibre 4g • protein 21g • salt 1.9g

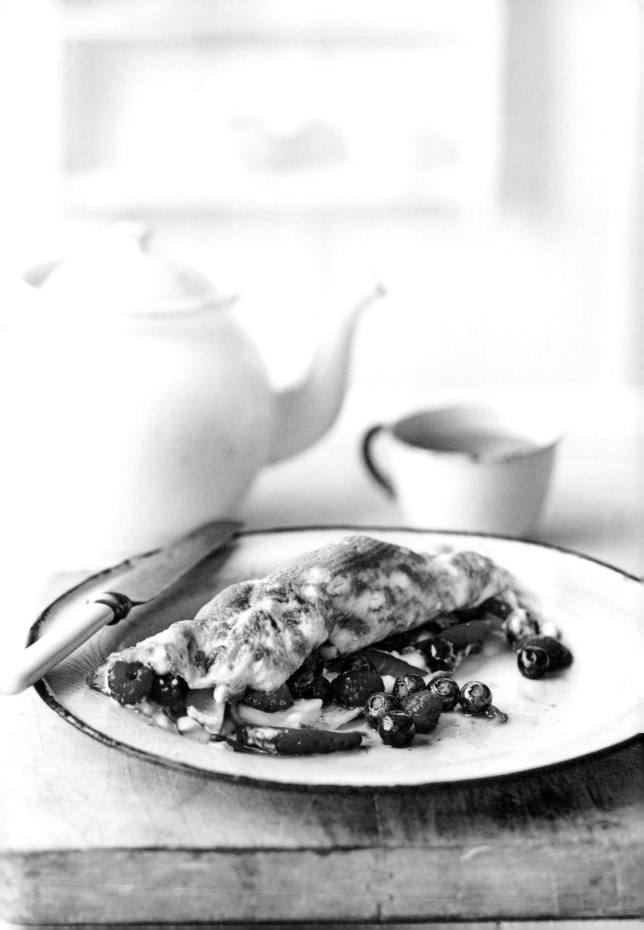

Grapefruit, Orange & Apricot Salad

Tangy and refreshing, this salad would make a great salad as part of breakfast as well as a reviving snack.

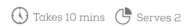 Takes 10 mins   Serves 2

- 1 grapefruit
- 2 oranges
- 2 fresh apricots, stoned and sliced or 4 canned halves in natural juice

1 First segment the grapefruit and oranges. One by one, cut a little horizontal slice from the top and bottom of each fruit so that they can sit flat on a board. Using a small, sharp knife, cut off the peel and pith in downward strokes, following the curve of the fruit. Work your way round until all the peel is removed.
2 Hold the fruit over a bowl to catch the juice and then cut free each segment by carefully slicing between the membranes to release it. Put the segments into the bowl of juice and gently stir in the apricot slices.

BENEFITS vegan • low fat • vit C • 2 of 5 a day • gluten free
PER SERVING 67 kcals • fat 0g • saturates 0g • carbs 13g • sugars 13g • fibre 4g • protein 2g • salt 0g

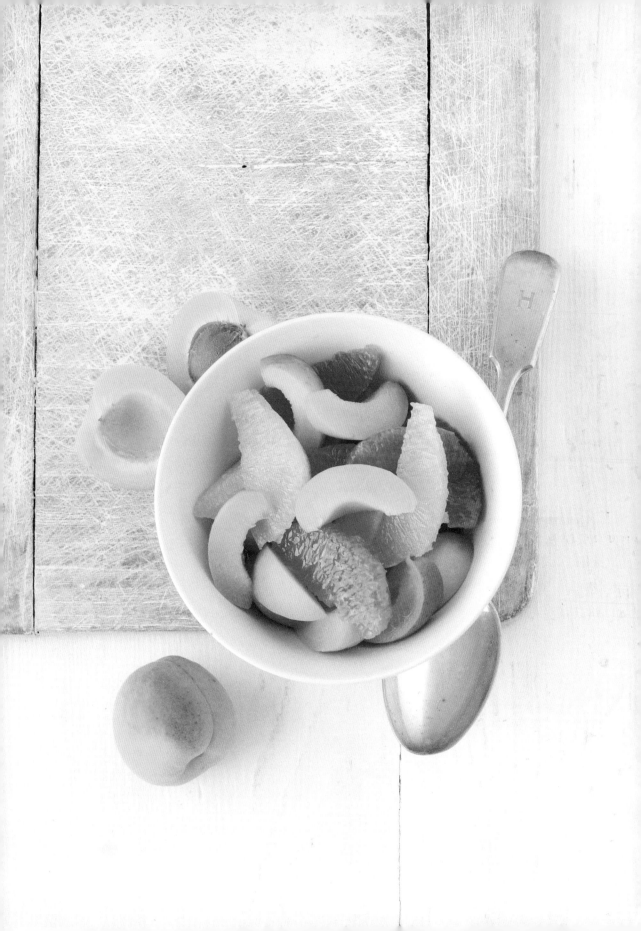

Instant Berry Banana Slush

This couldn't be simpler and is surprisingly creamy even though it doesn't contain dairy.

🕐 Takes 5 mins   ◔ Serves 4

- 2 ripe bananas
- 200g/7oz frozen berry mix (blackberries, raspberries and currants)

1 Slice the bananas into a bowl and add the frozen berry mix. Blitz with a stick blender to make a slushy ice and serve straight away in 2 glasses with spoons.

BENEFITS vegan • low fat • vit c • 1 of 5 a day • gluten free
PER SERVING 119 kcals • fat 0.4g • saturates 0.1g • carbs 24g • sugars 22g • fibre 5g • protein 2g • salt 0g

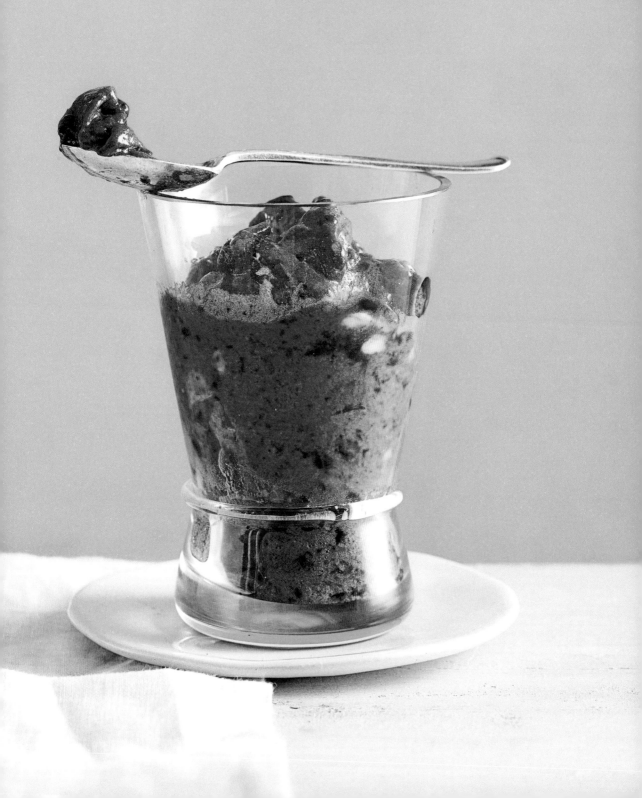

Minty Pineapple Smoothie

There's more to smoothies than just fruit - this dairy-free green blend contains spinach, oats, linseeds and cashew nuts, too. Use canned pineapple in fruit juice if more convenient than preparing a fresh one.

🕐 Takes 10 mins   ◔ Serves 2

- 200g/7oz pineapple, peeled, cored and cut into chunks
- a few mint leaves
- 50g/2oz baby spinach leaves
- 25g/1oz porridge oats
- 2 tbsp linseeds
- handful unsalted cashew nuts
- fresh lime juice, to taste

1 Put all the ingredients in a blender with 200ml/7fl oz water and process until smooth. If it's too thick, add more water (up to 400ml/14fl oz) until you get the right mix.

BENEFITS vegan • 1 of 5 a day
PER SERVING 177 kcals • fat 8g • saturates 19g • carbs 19g • sugars 11g • fibre 4g • protein 6g • salt 0.1g

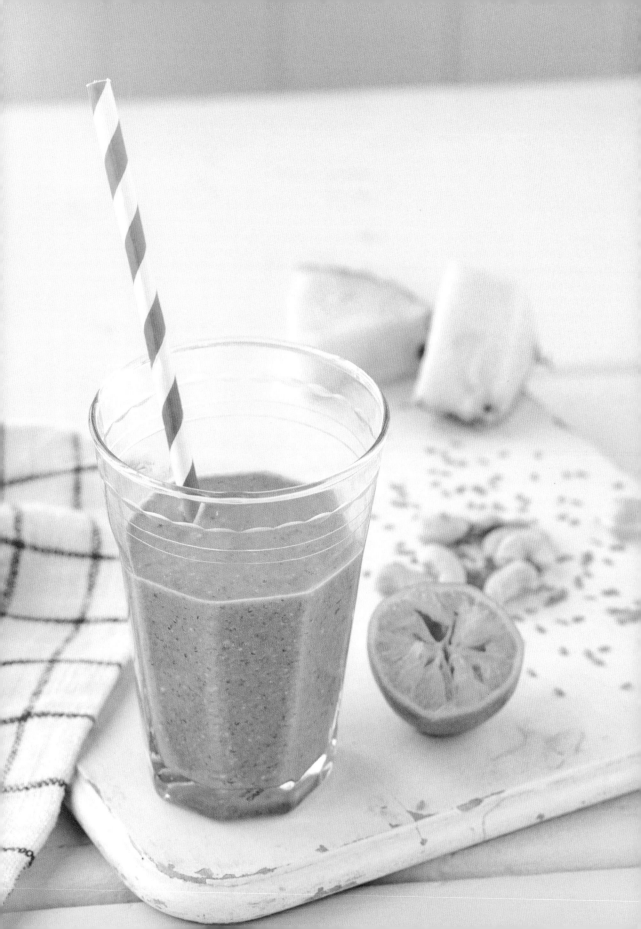

Sunshine Smoothie

If you have a juicer, you can make your own carrot juice for this smoothie.

Takes 5 mins   Serves 2-3

- 500ml/18fl oz carrot juice, chilled
- 200g/7oz pineapple (chopped fresh or canned in natural juice)
- 2 bananas, broken into chunks
- small piece of ginger, peeled
- 25g/1oz unsalted cashew nuts
- juice 1 lime

1 Put the ingredients in a blender and whizz until smooth. Drink straight away or pour into a bottle to drink on the go. Will keep in the fridge for a day.

BENEFITS vegan • low fat • 1 of 5 a day • gluten free
PER SERVING (3) 171 kcals • fat 4g • saturates 1g • carbs 30g • sugars 27g • fibre 3g • protein 3g • salt 0.2g

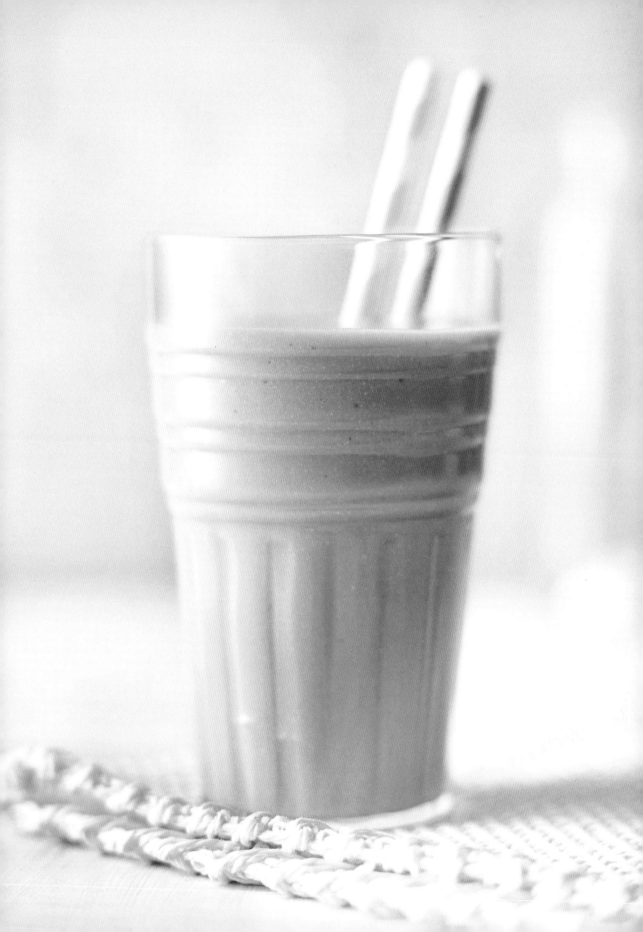

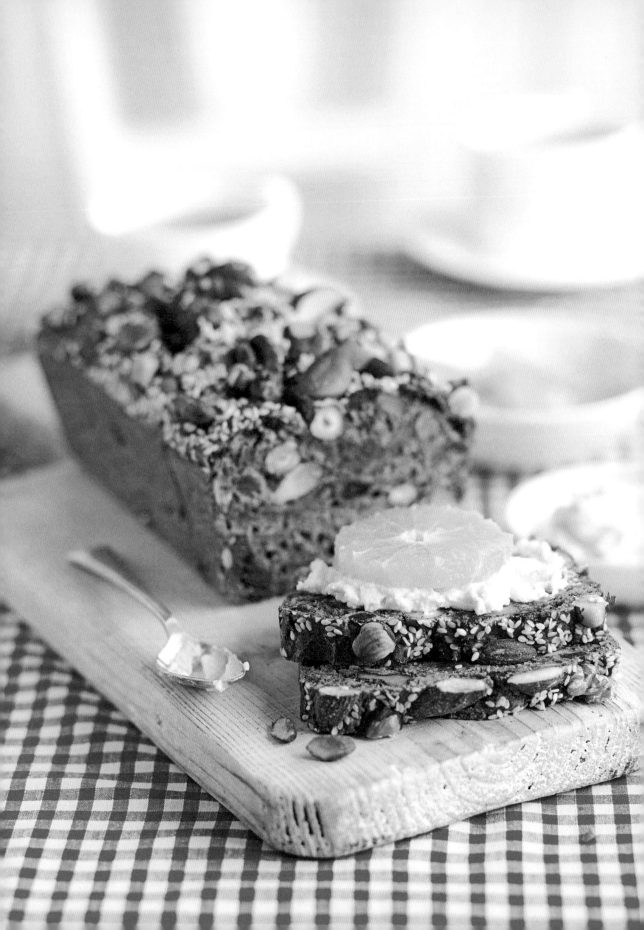

Chapter 5

BETTER-FOR-YOU BAKES, CAKES & DESSERTS

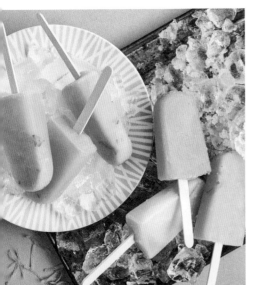
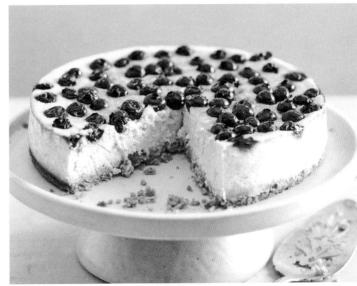
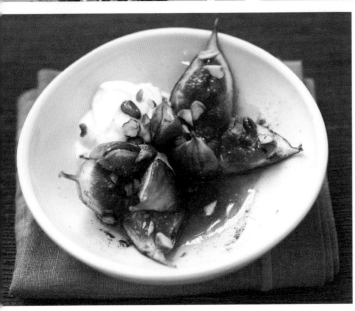
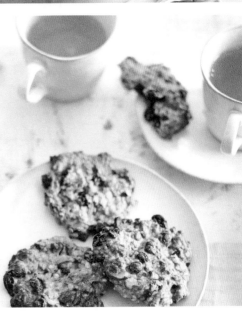

Home bakes

If you want to avoid excess sugar, unhealthy fats, salt, preservatives or emulsifiers, the answer is to do some home baking.

In this chapter you will find some healthy staples like breads and flatbreads along with plenty of healthier-for-you cakes and desserts. After all, a healthy, balanced diet is one that is followed for the long-term, so it's important that it incorporates social occasions when you see friends as well as the occasional treat.

While we do need some sugar in our diet to fuel our muscles and keep our brain on an even keel, we get plenty of what our body needs in the form of glucose, from the starchy carbs we eat. Foods like rice, bread and potatoes are all fabulous sources of the energy we require to get us through the day – what's more, they supply the additional nutrients that our bodies need too. Sugar, on the other hand, supplies empty calories – it gives us that fast kick of energy that is quickly followed by a crash and the associated irritability, tiredness and need for another sugar fix, which is why we need to restrict the amount we eat.

With this in mind many of our sweet bakes, cakes and desserts focus on sugars that release their energy slowly whilst also contributing useful amounts of fibre from wholemeal flour and nuts, 'good for you' fats and protein. Rather than turning to artificial sweeteners, instead of sugar we've used fresh and dried fruits, like sultanas, figs and raisins, as well as fresh apples, berries and banana. There are also some sweeter tasting vegetables like carrots and sweet potatoes – why not try our Lighter spiced carrot cake on page 278.

In some of our baking recipes we've used black strap molasses or black treacle because it helps to give bakes a distinctive flavour. Unlike refined sugar, black treacle supplies sweetness as well as valuable minerals including bone-building calcium, energising iron and B vitamins for the nervous system. However, we have occasionally used small amounts of maple syrup too. Don't think that's a licence to add it to all your recipes, we have been sparing as it is still sugar and will disrupt your blood sugar levels – what's more, it's the type of 'free' sugar we are advised to cut back on. However, it is a useful source of minerals including the immune-supportive mineral zinc and protective compounds called polyphenols, so it is better than other sweeteners like agave nectar or refined sugar.

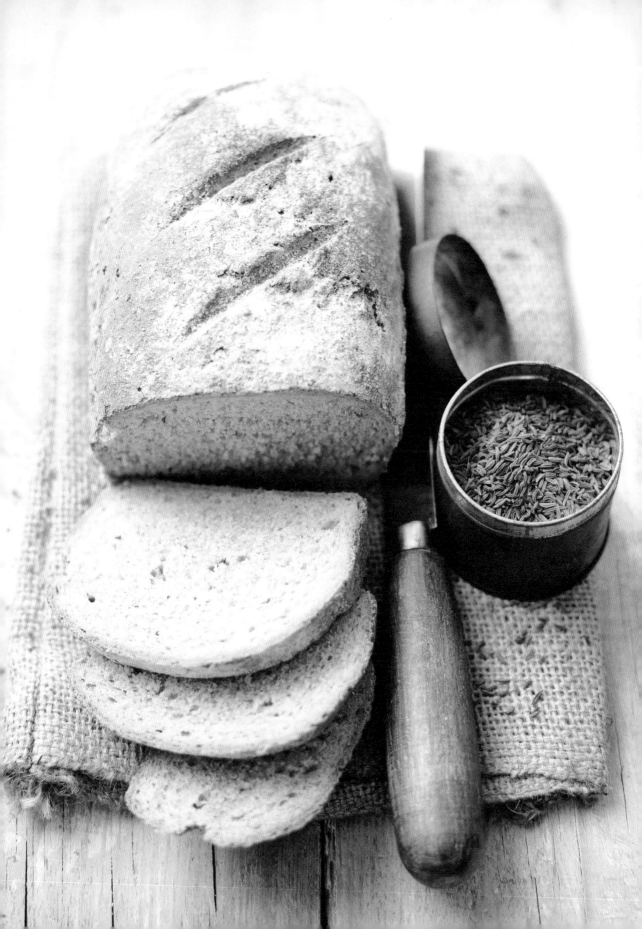

Flowerpot Loaves

Clay flowerpots need to be treated to stop the bread from sticking. To do this, generously brush the pots with oil and bake at 200C/180C fan/gas 4 for 1 hr. Remove from the oven, then wash and dry before using.

🕐 Takes 50 mins, plus rising   ◔ Makes 5

- 500g/12oz strong wholemeal or granary flour
- 7g sachet fast-action yeast
- 1 tsp salt
- 2 tbsp olive or rapeseed oil, plus extra for the flower pots
- 1 tbsp honey
- a little milk or oil for brushing

PLUS ANY OF THESE TOPPINGS
- 1 tbsp pumpkin, sunflower, sesame or poppy seeds
- 4 tbsp grated cheddar or crumbled feta cheese
- 1 tbsp chopped rosemary, thyme, oregano, chives or basil
- 1 tbsp chopped olives
- ½ tsp chilli flakes

YOU WILL ALSO NEED
- 5 small, clean clay flowerpots

1 Tip the flour, yeast and salt into a large bowl. Pour in 300ml warm water, the olive oil and honey. Mix with a wooden spoon until the mixture clumps together, then tip out onto a work surface. Use your hands to stretch and knead the dough for about 10 mins, or until it's smooth and springy. Add a little extra flour if the dough feels too sticky.

2 Brush the flowerpots with oil and line the sides with baking parchment. Divide the dough into 5 pieces and shape into smooth balls. Place one ball of dough into each flowerpot and cover with cling film. Leave in a warm place for 1 hr to rise.

3 Heat oven to 200C/180C fan/gas 6. When the dough has doubled in size, remove the cling film from the pots and gently brush the dough with a little milk or oil. Sprinkle with your choice of topping.

4 Place the pots on a baking tray then bake for 20-25 mins until risen and golden. The pots will be very hot, so be careful when removing from the oven. Leave to cool for 10 mins before turning out and eating.

BENEFITS vegetarian
PER SLICE 435 kcals, fat 8g, saturates 1g, carbs 47g, sugars 4g, fibre 3g protein 13g, salt 1g

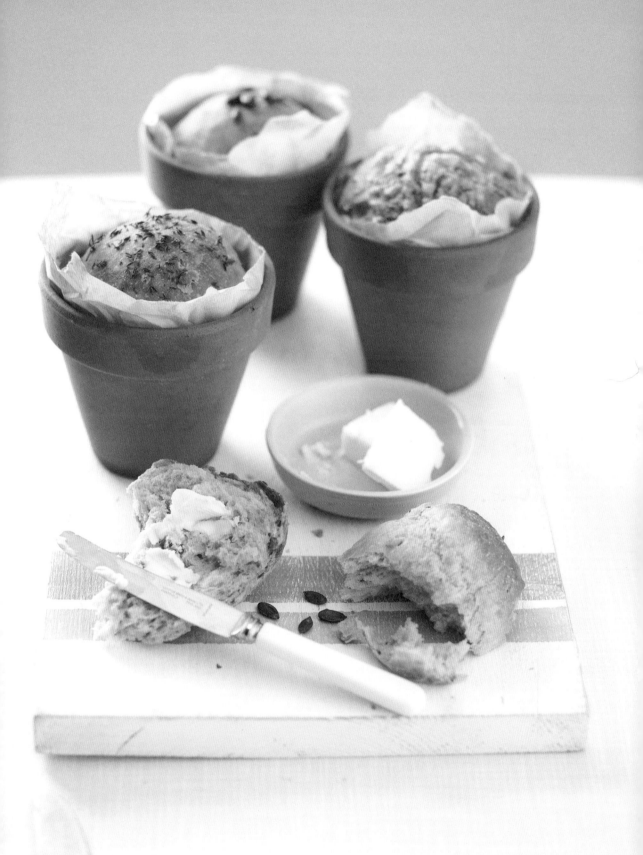

Seeded Wholemeal Loaf

Some 100% wholemeal loaves can be a bit heavy, so this has spelt flour added to lighten the texture. The seeds add a lovely texture, while the black treacle, used instead of refined sugar, gives it a rich flavour and golden colour.

Takes 1 hour 20 mins, plus proving   Cuts into 10-12 slices

- 400g/14oz strong wholemeal bread flour
- 100g/4oz spelt flour
- 7g sachet fast-action dried yeast
- 1 tbsp black treacle
- rapeseed oil, for greasing
- 50g/2oz mixed seeds (try pumpkin, sunflower, poppy and linseeds) (optional)
- 1 egg yolk, loosened with a fork

1 Combine both flours in a large bowl with the yeast and 1 tsp fine salt. Mix the treacle with 250ml/9fl oz warm water until well combined. Stir into the flour to make a slightly sticky dough. If you need to add more water, splash it in 1 tbsp at a time.

2 Knead the dough on a lightly floured surface for 10 mins (or in a tabletop mixer for 5-7 mins). Your dough should be smooth and elastic when it's ready. Place the dough in a lightly oiled bowl, flip the dough over to coat it in oil, then cover with a sheet of oiled cling film. Leave in a warm place until doubled in size – this will take about 1 hour. Alternatively, you can leave the dough to prove overnight in the fridge. Take it out of the fridge on the day of baking and leave it for at least 45 mins so it comes to room temperature.

3 Lightly oil a 900g/2lb loaf tin. Knead the dough again for 3-5 mins to knock out the air bubbles – add most of the seeds and work these into the dough as you knead. Shape the dough into an oval roughly the same length as your tin. Place in the tin and leave to prove, covered with oiled cling film, for 30-45 mins until it has nearly doubled in size again. Heat oven to 200C/180C fan/gas 6.

4 Glaze the top of the loaf with the egg yolk and sprinkle over the remaining seeds. Bake in the oven for 40-45 mins until golden brown – if you tip the loaf out of the tin and tap the bottom, it should sound hollow. Leave to cool on a wire rack for at least 30 mins before slicing.

BENEFITS *vegetarian*
PER SLICE (12) 173 kcals • fat 3g • saturates 1g • carbs 27g • sugars 2g • fibre 5g • protein 7g • salt 0.4g

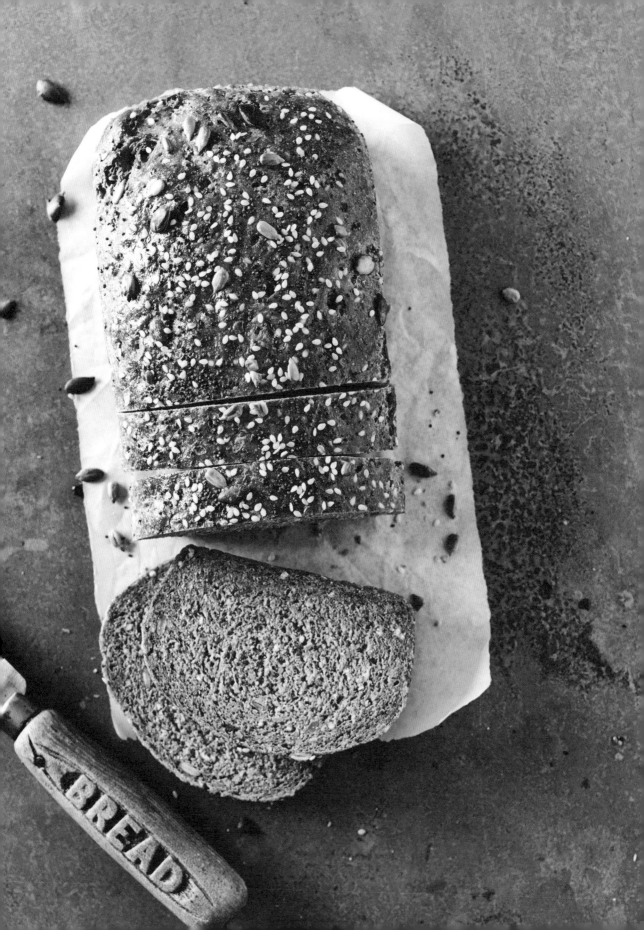

Rye Bread

Caraway seeds add a slightly aniseed hit to this bread, so just leave them out if you prefer. Rye flour initiates a lower blood sugar response than wheat, making it a better choice if you struggle to manage your blood sugar levels.

🕐 Takes 50 minutes, plus proving   🕐 Cuts into 8 slices

- 200g/7oz rye flour, plus extra for dusting
- 200g/7oz strong wholemeal bread flour
- 7g sachet fast-action dried yeast
- ½ tsp salt
- 1 tbsp clear honey
- rapeseed oil, for greasing
- 1 tsp caraway seed (optional)

1 Tip the flours, yeast and salt into a bowl. In a jug, mix the honey with 250ml/9floz warm water, pour the liquid into the bowl and mix to form a dough. Rye flour can be quite dry and absorbs lots of water. If the dough looks too dry, add more warm water until you have a soft dough. Tip out onto a lightly floured work surface and knead for 10 mins until smooth. Rye contains less gluten than white flour so the dough will not feel as springy as a conventional white loaf. Place the dough in a well-oiled bowl, cover with cling film and leave to rise in a warm place for 1-2 hours or until roughly doubled in size. Dust a 900g/2lb loaf tin with flour.

2 Tip the dough back onto a lightly floured work surface and knead briefly to knock out any air bubbles. If using caraway seeds, work these into the dough. Shape into a smooth oval loaf and pop into your tin. Cover the tin with oiled cling film and leave to rise somewhere warm for a further 1-1 hour 30 mins, or until doubled in size.

3 Heat oven to 220C/200C fan/gas 7. Remove the cling film and dust the surface of the loaf with rye flour. Slash a few incisions on an angle, then bake for 30 mins until dark brown and hollow sounding when tapped. Transfer to a wire cooling rack and leave to cool for at least 20 mins before serving.

BENEFITS *vegetarian • low fat • fibre*
PER SLICE *187 kcals • fat 1g • saturates 0.1g • carbs 36g • sugars 2g • fibre 7g • protein 6g • salt 0.3g*

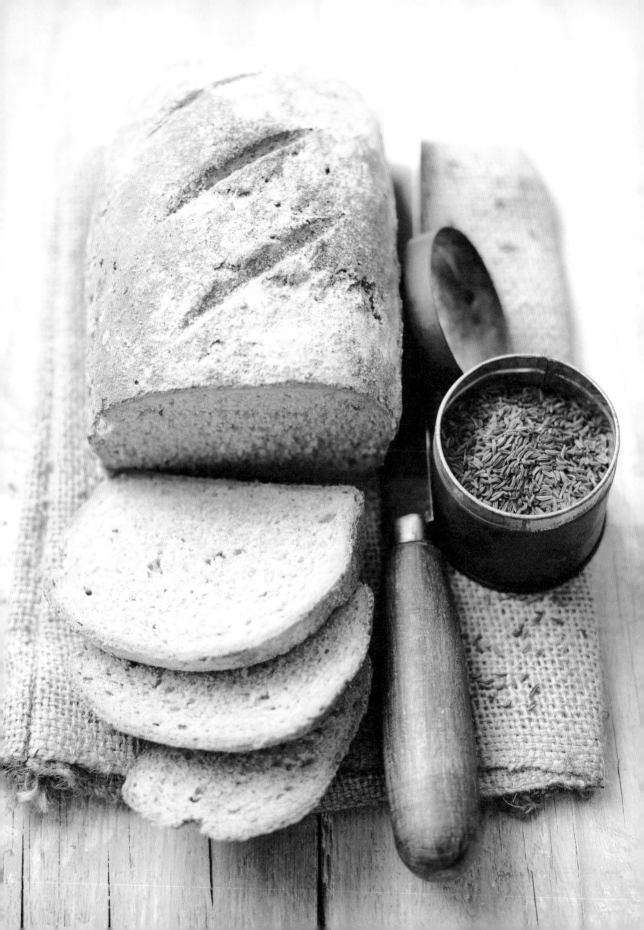

Wholemeal Flatbreads

These flatbreads are a doddle – simply make a large batch and freeze them for later in the week. Shop-bought flatbreads are likely to contain preservatives and emulsifiers, so our homemade version are a healthier choice.

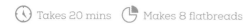 Takes 20 mins   Makes 8 flatbreads

- 350g/12oz wholemeal flour, plus extra for dusting
- 4 tsp rapeseed oil

1 Put the flour in a medium bowl and rub in the oil with your fingertips. Stir in 225ml/8fl oz warm water, mix thoroughly, then knead until the dough feels smooth and elastic.

2 Put the dough onto a lightly floured surface and divide into 8 balls. Sprinkle the work surface with a little more flour and roll out 1 of the balls very thinly, using a floured rolling pin, to around 22cm/9in in diameter. Turn the dough regularly and sprinkle with a little more flour if it begins to stick. Set aside and make the other flatbreads in the same way. If making ahead, freeze before cooking.

3 Put a medium non-stick frying pan over a high heat and, once hot, add 1 of the flatbreads. Cook for about 30 secs, then turn over and cook on the other side for 30 secs. Press the flatbread with a spatula while cooking to encourage it to puff up and cook inside – it should be lightly browned in patches and look fairly dry, without being crisp. Repeat with the remaining flatbreads, keeping them warm by wrapping in a clean tea towel until needed.

BENEFITS vegan
PER FLATBREAD 168 kcals • fat 2g • saturates 0g • carbs 27g • sugars 1g • fibre 5g • protein 6g • salt 0g

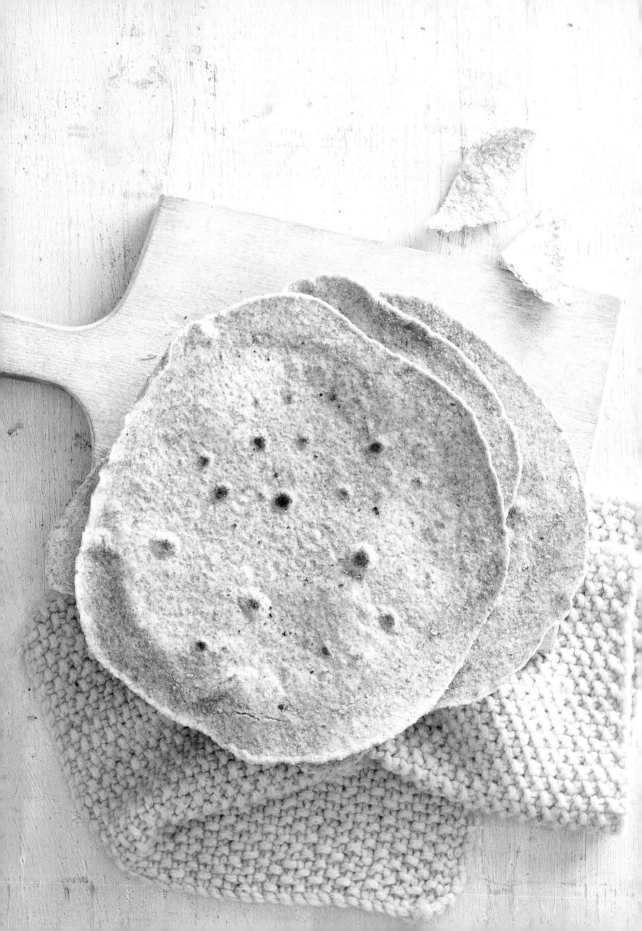

Fig & Nut Seed Bread

Keep this in the fridge, or portion the slices for the freezer for a great breakfast when you are short of time. Top with ricotta or soft cheese and fresh fruit as an alternative to butter.

 Takes 1 hour 30 mins   Cuts into 16 slices

- 400ml/14fl oz hot strong black tea
- 100g/4oz dried figs, hard stalks removed, thinly sliced
- 140g/5oz sultanas
- 50g/2oz porridge oats
- 200g/7oz self-raising wholemeal flour
- 1 tsp baking powder
- 100g/4oz mixed nuts (almonds, walnuts, Brazils, hazelnuts), plus 50g/2oz for the top
- 1 tbsp each golden linseeds and sesame seeds, plus 2 tsp sesame to sprinkle
- 25g/1oz pumpkin seeds
- 1 large egg

TO SERVE
- 25g/1oz ricotta for spreading
- 1 thick slice of orange or green apple

1 Heat oven to 170C/150C fan/gas 3. Pour the tea into a large bowl and stir in the figs, sultanas and oats. Set aside to soak while you get on with the rest of the loaf.
2 Line the base and sides of a 900g/2lb loaf tin with baking parchment. Mix the flour, baking powder, 100g/4oz nuts and the seeds. Beat the egg into the cooled fruit mixture, then stir the dried ingredients in to the wet. Pile into the tin, then level the top and scatter with the remaining nuts and sesame seeds.
3 Bake for 1 hour, then cover the top with foil and bake for 15 mins more until a skewer inserted into the centre of the loaf comes out clean. Remove from the tin to cool, but leave the paper on until cold. Serve sliced spread with ricotta rather than butter, which is lower in fat and higher in protein, and fruit. It will keep in the fridge for a month.

BENEFITS vegetarian
PER SLICE 175 kcals • fat 7g • saturates 1g • carbs 20g • sugars 10g • fibre 3g • protein 6g • salt 0.1g

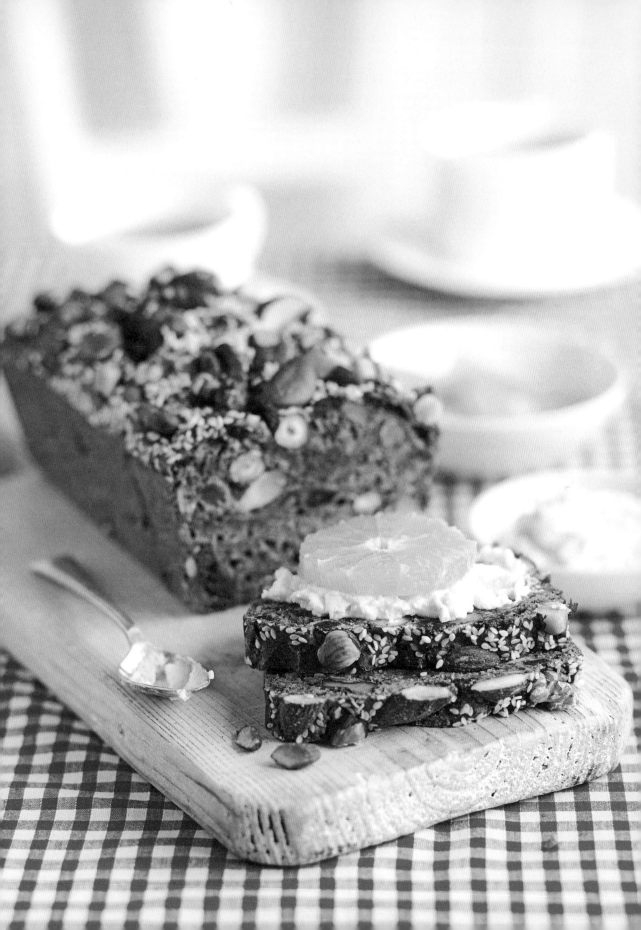

Oaty Hazelnut Cookies

These have a soft, slightly chewy texture as they contain apple instead of sugar. They're packed with hazelnuts, which are a good source of the vitamins and minerals needed for healthy hair, skin and nails.

🕐 Takes 45 mins   🥧 Makes 9 cookies

- 50g/2oz butter, plus a little for greasing
- 2 tbsp maple syrup
- 1 eating apple, unpeeled and coarsely grated (you need 85g/3oz)
- 1 tsp ground cinnamon
- 50g/2oz raisins
- 50g/2oz porridge oats
- 50g/2oz spelt flour
- 40g/1½oz unblanched hazelnuts, cut into chunky slices
- 1 egg

1 Heat oven to 180C/160C fan/gas 4 and lightly grease a non-stick baking tray (or line a normal baking tray with baking parchment). Tip the butter and syrup into a small non-stick pan and melt together, then add the apple and cook, stirring, over a medium heat until it softens, about 6-7 mins. Stir in the cinnamon and raisins.

2 Mix the oats, spelt flour and hazelnuts in a bowl, pour in the apple mixture, then add the egg and beat everything together really well.

3 Spoon onto the baking tray, well spaced apart to make 9 mounds, then gently press into discs. Bake for 18-20 mins until golden, then cool on a wire rack. Will keep for 3 days in an airtight container or 6 weeks in the freezer.

BENEFITS vegetarian
PER COOKIE 146 kcals • fat 8g • saturates 3g • carbs 15g • sugars 8g • fibre 2g • protein 2g • salt 0.1g

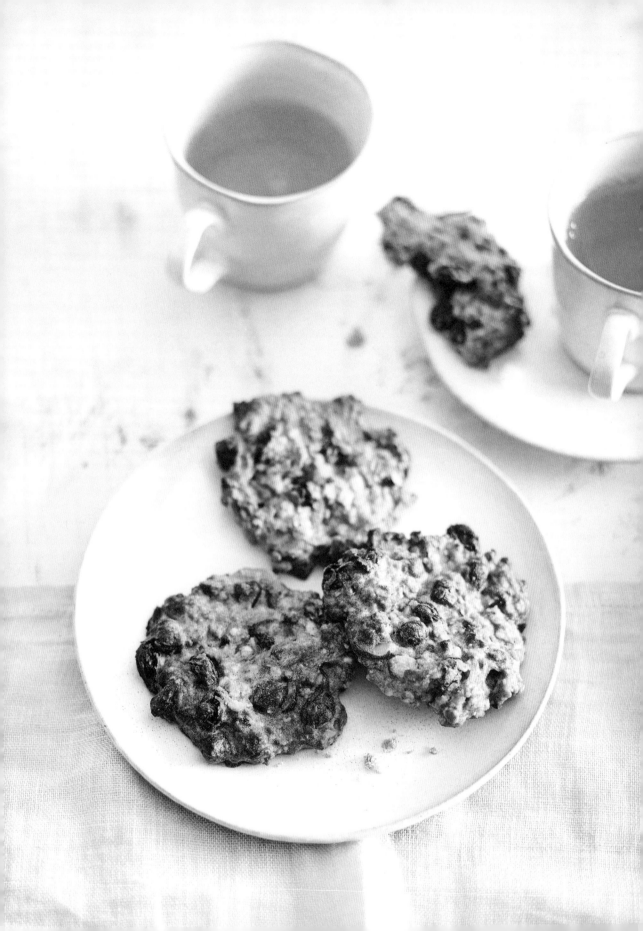

Lighter Spiced Carrot Cake

Who doesn't love carrot cake? This moist, classic tray bake uses sweet potato as well as carrots for their natural sweetness, so we can reduce the amount of added sugar.

🕐 Takes 1 hour 🥧 Cuts into 15 squares

- 100ml/3½fl oz rapeseed oil, plus a little extra for greasing
- 300g/11oz wholemeal flour
- 2 tsp baking powder
- 1 tsp bicarbonate of soda
- 1 tbsp mixed spice
- 1 tsp ground cinnamon
- 140g/5oz carrots, grated
- 140g/5oz sweet potatoes, peeled and grated
- 200g/7oz sultanas
- 3 large eggs
- 2 tbsp maple syrup
- 1 tsp vanilla extract
- juice 2 oranges

FOR THE ICING
- 175g/6oz soft cheese
- 3-4 tbsp live bio yogurt
- 1 tbsp maple syrup
- zest ½ orange

1 Heat oven to 180C/160C fan/gas 4. Grease and line a 20 x 30cm/8 x 12in traybake tin with baking parchment. Mix together the flour, baking powder, bicarb and spices in a big mixing bowl. Stir in the grated carrots, sweet potatoes and sultanas. In a jug, whisk together the eggs, rapeseed oil, syrup, vanilla and orange juice. Tip the wet ingredients into the dry and stir to combine, then scrape into the tin. Bake for 25-30 mins until a skewer poked in comes out clean. Cool in the tin.

2 Once cool, make the icing. Beat the cheese with the yogurt, syrup and orange zest. Spread all over the cake and slice into squares to eat.

BENEFITS vegetarian
PER SQUARE 249 kcals • fat 11g • saturates 3g • carbs 30g •. sugars 15g • fibre 3g • protein 6g • salt 0.5g

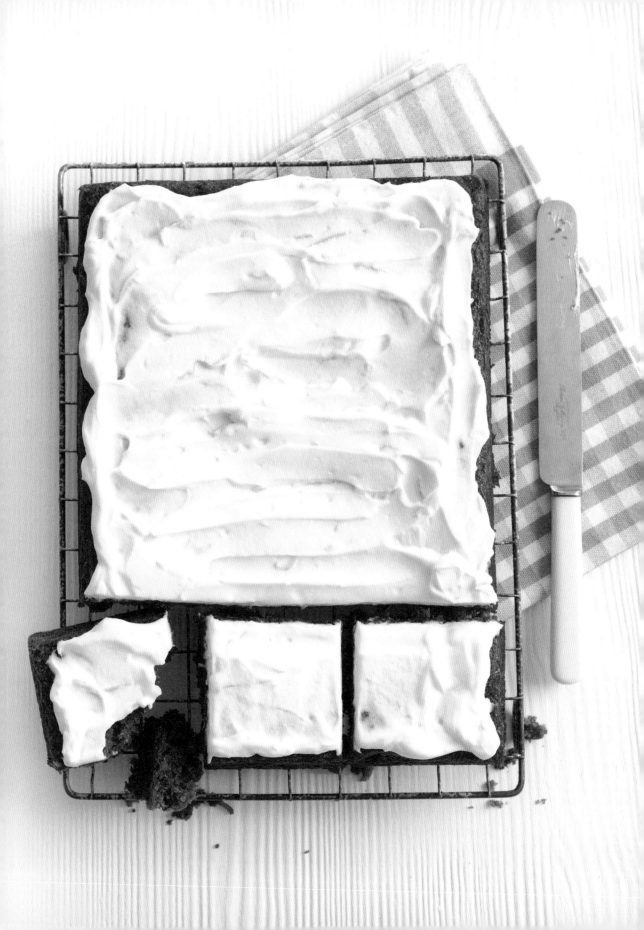

Sugar-free Banana Cake

The natural sweetness of fruit means no added sugar is needed in this wholefood banana bread. Delicious served hot or cold.

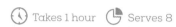 Takes 1 hour   Serves 8

- 125g/4½oz self-raising wholemeal flour
- ½ tsp baking powder
- 2 tsp ground cinnamon
- 75g/3oz sultanas
- 50g/2oz butter
- 2 tsp vanilla essence
- 1 egg
- 1 tbsp milk
- 3 ripe bananas, mashed

1 Preheat the oven to 180C/160C fan/ gas mark 4. Grease and line a 450g/1lb loaf tin with baking parchment.

2 Weigh the flour, baking powder, cinnamon and sultanas into a bowl and mix with a wooden spoon. Then weigh the butter, vanilla essence, egg, milk and mashed bananas and put into another bowl or jug and mix with a small balloon whisk or fork. Pour the 'wet' banana mixture into the 'dry' flour mixture and combine thoroughly with a wooden spoon.

3 Pour the cake mixture into the prepared tin and bake for 30-40 mins or until a skewer inserted in the middle comes out clean. Remove from the oven, allow to cool in the tin for 10 mins, then turn out.

BENEFITS vegetarian
PER SERVING 174 kcals • fat 6g • saturates 4g • carbs 24g • sugars 13g • fibre 3g • protein 3g • salt0.2g

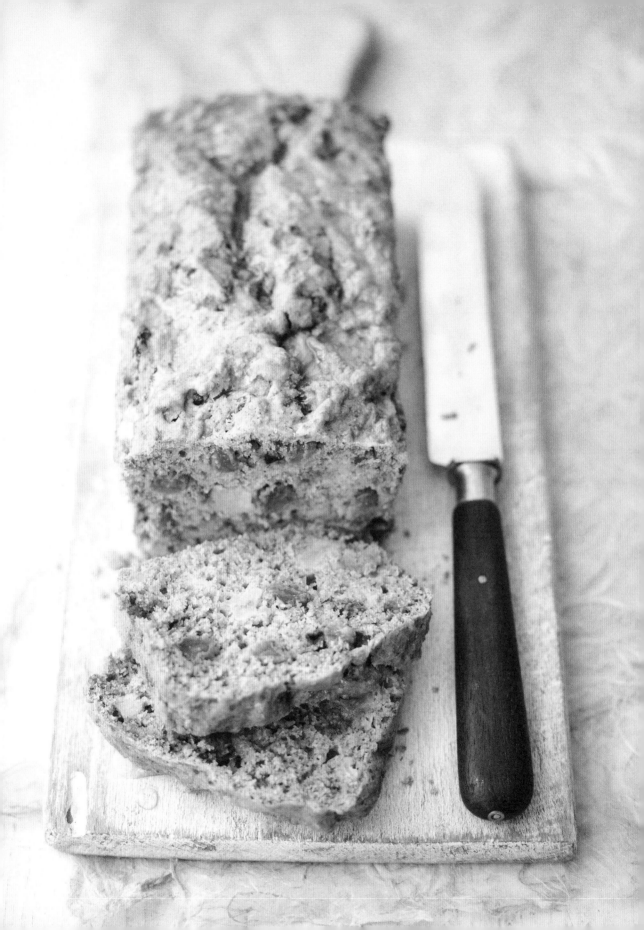

Bread Pudding

This healthier version of an all-time favourite is packed full of flavour – we've used dried fruit for sweetness and what's more, it counts towards your 5 a day.

🕐 Takes 1 hour 25 mins   ◔ Cuts into 9-12 squares

- 400g/14oz wholemeal bread, preferably homemade (page 268)
- 400g/14oz mixed dried fruit
- 2 tbsp mixed spice
- 400ml/14fl oz milk
- 2 large eggs, beaten
- zest and juice 1 small orange
- 75g/3½oz butter, melted, plus extra for greasing

1 Tear the bread into a large mixing bowl and add the fruit and spice. Pour in the milk, then stir or scrunch through your fingers to mix everything well and completely break up the bread. Add the eggs and orange zest and juice. Stir well, then set aside for 15 mins to soak.

2 Heat oven to 180C/160C fan/gas 4. Butter and line the base of a 20cm/8in non-stick square cake tin (not one with a loose base). Stir the melted butter into the pudding mixture, and tip into the tin. Bake for 1 hour until firm and golden. Turn out of the tin and strip off the paper. Cut into squares and serve warm or cold.

BENEFITS vegetarian • 1 of 5 a day
PER SERVING (9) 255 kcals • fat 8g • saturates 4g • carbs 37g • sugars 24g • fibre 3g • protein 7g • salt 0.6g

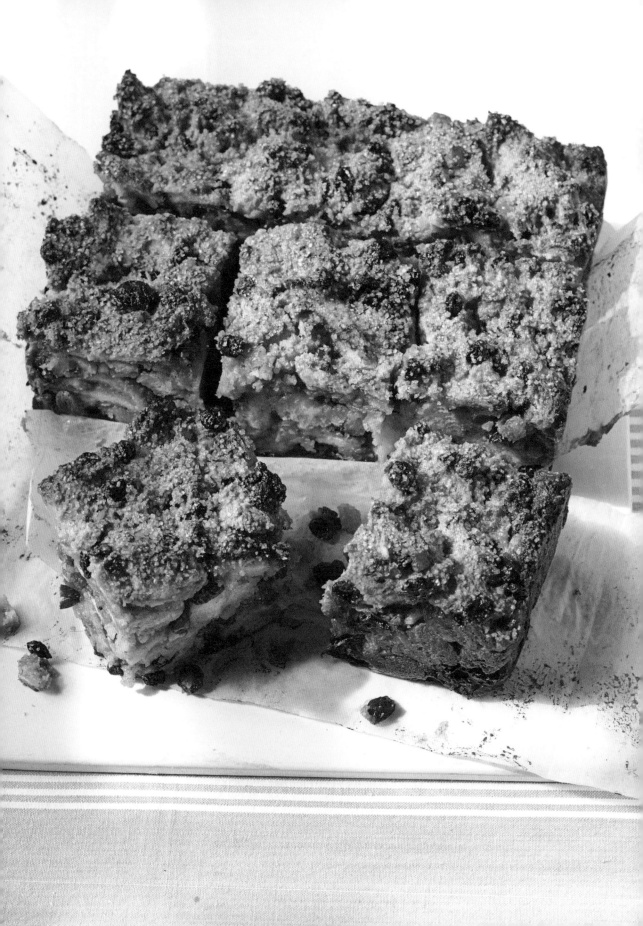

Cinnamon Crêpes with Nut Butter, Banana & Raspberries

Our nutritious batter is topped off with fresh fruit and a dollop of protein-packed nut butter, making a well-balanced, yet delicious pud.

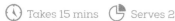 Takes 15 mins Serves 2

- 75g/2½fl oz wholemeal flour
- 1 tsp ground cinnamon
- 1 egg
- 225ml/8fl oz milk
- 1 tsp rapeseed oil
- 2 tbsp Almond butter (page 240)
- 1 banana, sliced
- 140g/5oz raspberries
- lemon wedges

1 Tip the flour into a large mixing bowl with the cinnamon. Add the egg and milk, and whisk vigorously until you have a smooth pouring consistency.
2 Place a non-stick frying pan over a medium heat and add a little of the oil. When the oil starts to heat, wipe most of it away with kitchen paper. Once the pan is hot, pour a small amount of the batter into the centre of the pan and swirl it to the sides of the pan in a thin layer. Leave to cook, untouched, for about 2 mins. When it is brown underneath, turn over and cook for 1 min more.
3 Transfer to a warm plate and cover with foil to keep warm. Repeat with the remaining batter. Divide the warm pancakes between 2 plates and serve with the nut butter, banana, raspberries and lemon to assemble at the table.

BENEFITS vegetarian • fibre • calcium • vit C • folate • 1 of 5 a day
PER SERVING 395 kcals • fat 15g • saturates 3g • carbs 44g • sugars 18g • fibre 9g • protein 16g • salt 0.2g

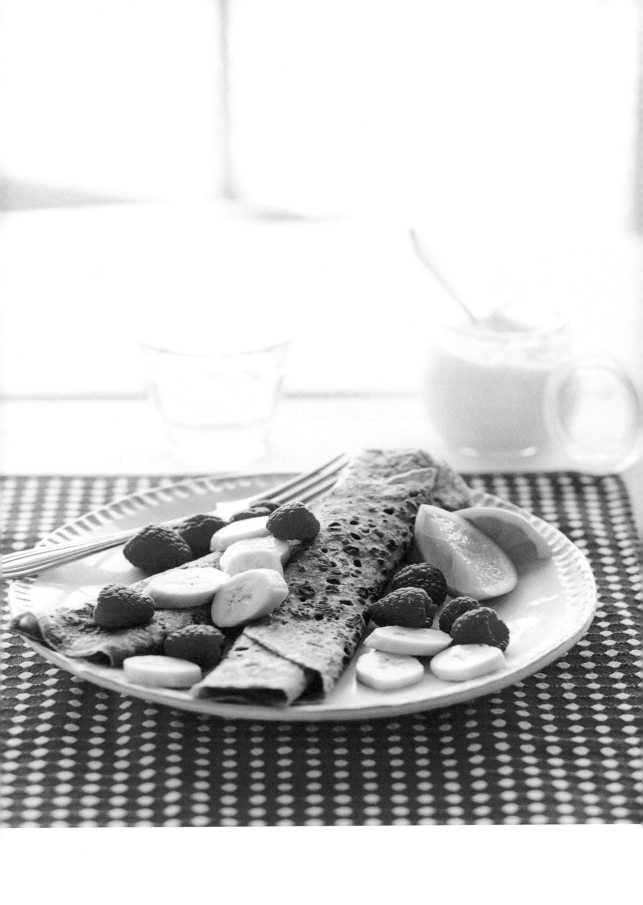

Baked Almond Banana & Blueberry Cheesecake

Sweetened with natural fruits and a small amount of maple syrup, this cheesecake combines ricotta and yogurt for a lower-fat, yet rich and creamy, texture. Maple syrup is still a 'free' sugar – the type we need to cut back on – but it does contribute small amounts of nutrients like manganese, calcium and zinc, so is better to use than honey or agave syrup.

 Takes 1 hour 10 mins Serves 10

FOR THE BASE
- 50g/2oz butter, plus a little for greasing
- 1 tsp maple syrup
- 75g/3oz oatcakes, finely crushed to crumbs
- 40g/1½oz ground almonds

FOR THE TOPPING
- 2 ripe bananas
- 2 x 250g tubs ricotta
- 150g pot live bio yogurt
- 4 large eggs, beaten
- 2 tbsp maple syrup
- 2 tsp vanilla extract
- 2 tbsp ground almonds
- 140g/5oz blueberries

1 Heat oven to 180C/160C fan/gas 4 and lightly grease a 20cm/8in round non-stick springform cake tin. Melt the butter and syrup in a pan, then stir in the oatcakes and almonds until well mixed and coated. Press firmly into the base of the tin to make a compact layer, then bake for 10 mins. Remove from the oven and increase the temperature to 240C/220C fan/gas 9.

2 To make the filling, mash the bananas in a large bowl. Add the ricotta, yogurt, eggs, syrup, vanilla and almonds, and beat with a wooden spoon until everything is very well mixed. Pour onto the base, scatter over the blueberries and bake for 10 mins, then turn the oven down to 110C/90C fan/gas ¼ and cook for 30-35 mins more. It should still have a bit of wobble in the middle when you gently shake the tin. Turn off the oven and leave the cheesecake inside to cool and set. Chill before serving.

BENEFITS vegetarian
PER SERVING 265 kcals • fat 17g • saturates 8g • carbs 15g • sugars 10g • fibre 1g • protein 11g • salt 0.5g

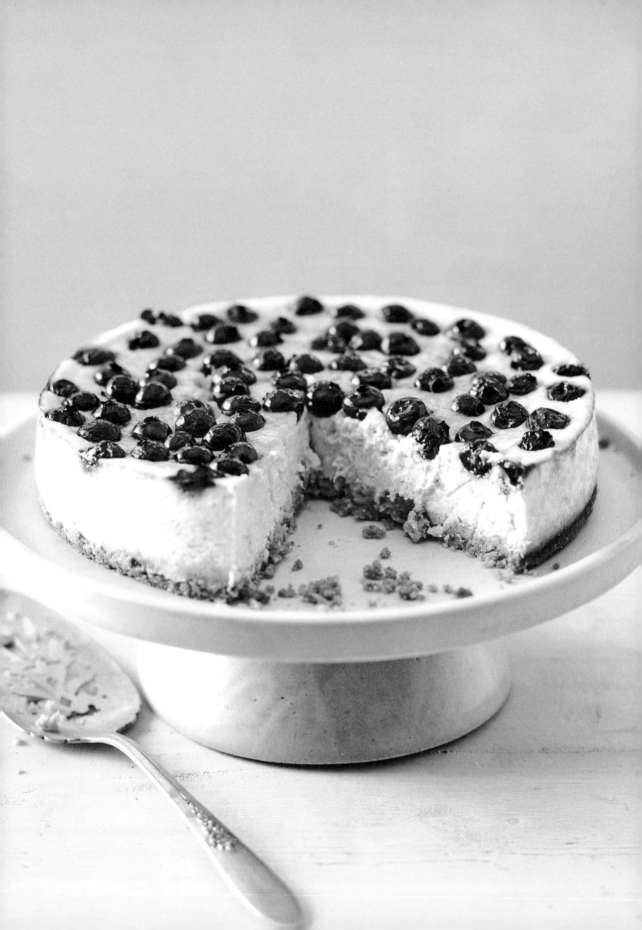

Sunshine Lollies

If you have a juicer use it instead of grating the carrots to extract their juice. Our sunshine lollies are an altogether more natural way to enjoy a little sweetness on a hot summer's day.

Takes 20 mins, plus overnight freezing   Makes 6 x 60ml/2½fl oz lollies

- 5 large carrots
- juice 3 large oranges, zest of 1
- 1 satsuma, peeled, then chopped (optional)

1 Finely grate the carrots and place in the middle of a clean tea towel. Gather up the towel, and squeeze the carrot juice into a jug, discarding the pulp. Add the orange juice and top up with a little cold water if needed to make up 360ml/12fl oz liquid.
2 Stir in the orange zest and satsuma pieces, if using. Pour into lolly moulds and freeze overnight.

BENEFITS vegan • low fat • gluten free
PER LOLLY 17 kcals • fat 0g • saturates 0g • carbs 4g • sugars 4g • fibre 0g • protein 0g • salt 0g

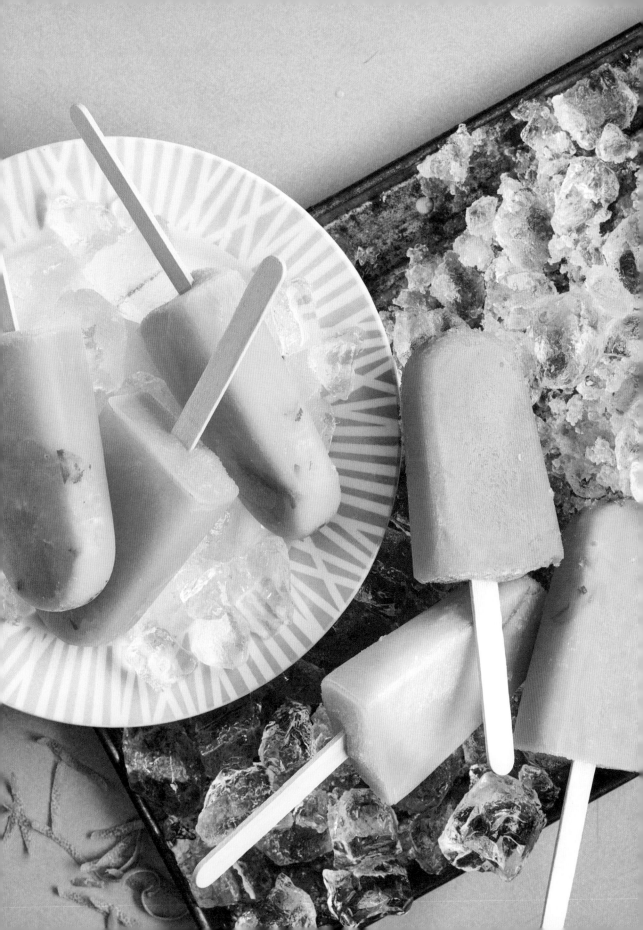

Creamy Avo Lollies

Amazingly versatile, avocados add delicious texture and creaminess to our sophisticated, grown-up lollies.

🕐 Takes 10 mins, plus overnight freezing   🕐 Makes 8 x 60ml/2½fl oz lollies

- 2 small ripe avocados, stoned and peeled
- juice 2 limes
- 250ml/9fl oz live bio yogurt
- 1 tsp vanilla extract
- 2 tbsp maple syrup

1 Tip all the ingredients into a food processor and blitz until smooth.
2 Spoon into lolly moulds and freeze overnight.

BENEFITS vegetarian • gluten free
PER LOLLY 89 kcals • fat 6g • saturates 2g • carbs 6g • sugars 5g • fibre 1g • protein 2g • salt 0.1g

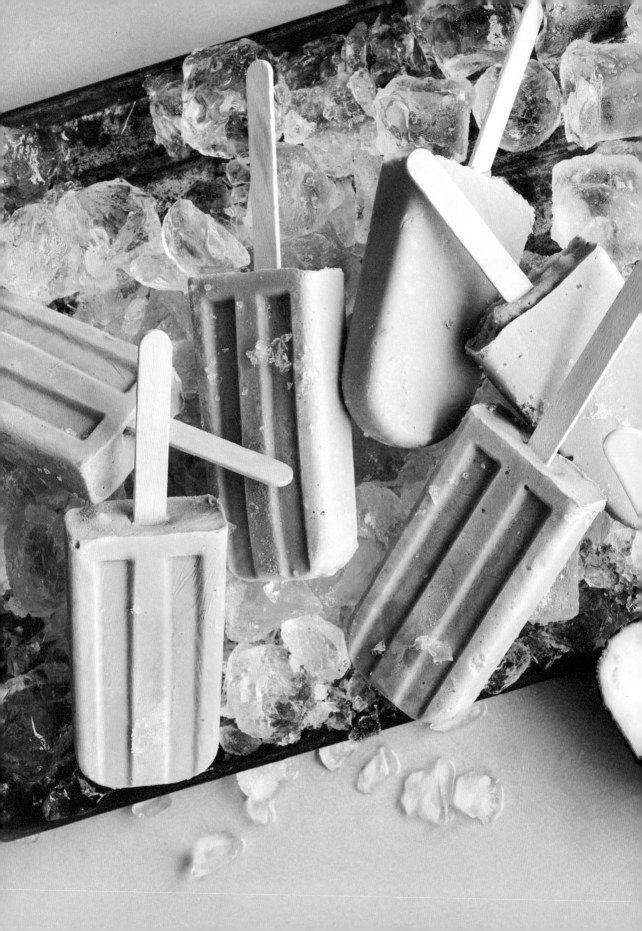

Blueberry & Coconut Frozen 'Cheesecake' Bars

Our 'cheesecake' bars are gluten and dairy free. They're so easy to make, store well and look impressive.

🕐 Takes 35 mins, plus chilling   🥧 Makes 10-12 bars

- 280g/10oz unsalted cashew nuts
- rapeseed oil, for greasing

FOR THE BASE
- 140g/5oz unsalted almonds
- 140g/5oz pitted dates

FOR THE 'CHEESECAKE' LAYER
- 100g/4oz coconut cream
- 2 tbsp coconut oil, melted
- 2 tbsp maple syrup
- 1 tsp vanilla extract
- juice ½ lemon

FOR THE TOPPING
- 140g/5oz blueberries, plus a handful
- 5 pitted dates

1 Soak the cashew nuts in boiling water for 10 mins, or overnight in cold water if you have time. Lightly oil a 20cm/8in square cake tin.
2 To make the base, whizz the unsalted almonds and pitted dates in a food processor until very finely chopped. Tip into the tin and press the mixture down, smoothing with the back of a spoon until evenly spread across the base. Put the tin in the freezer to firm up while you make the 'cheesecake' layer.
3 Drain the cashew nuts and put half in the food processor. Add the ingredients for the 'cheesecake' layer and blitz until smooth and creamy. Remove the tin from the freezer and spread the creamy mixture on top of the base. Return to the freezer for 30-40 mins until firm.
4 To make the topping, blend the 140g/5oz blueberries and the dates together with the remaining cashews in the food processor. Take the tin out of the freezer and spoon over the topping, then scatter over a handful of blueberries. Return to the freezer for at least 1 hour to firm up. Can be stored in the freezer for up to 2 months. Remove from the freezer 10 mins before serving, then slice into 10-12 bars and enjoy.

BENEFITS vegan • gluten free
PER BAR (12) 326 kcals • fat 21g • saturates 6g • carbs 23g • sugars 19g • fibre 3g • protein 8g • salt 0g

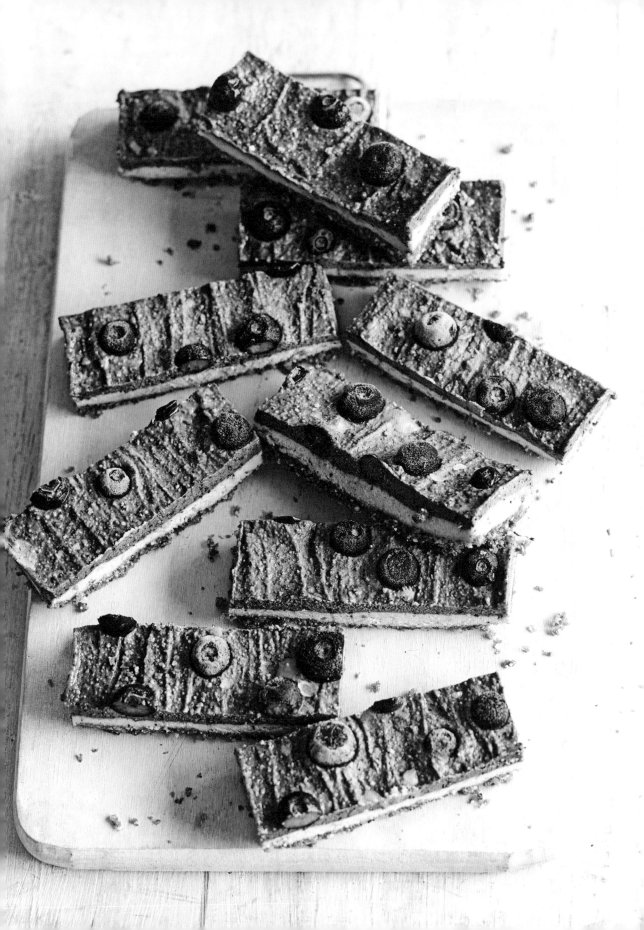

Bear's Chocolate Mousse

This is ridiculously quick to make. If you have an unexpected guest, it's guaranteed to be a winner!

🕐 Takes 5 mins, plus chilling   🥧 Serves 2

- 2 eggs
- 4 slightly heaped tbsp cacao powder
- 4 tbsp maple syrup
- 2 tbsp coconut oil, melted and cooled
- dash of vanilla essence

1 Put all the ingredients in a large bowl and mix with a whisk until smooth.
2 Divide into 2 ramekins and put in the fridge for at least 30 mins to set. Then serve – with a tiny spoon to make it last longer!

BENEFITS vegetarian • gluten free,
PER SERVING 350 kcals • fat 18g • saturates 12g • carbs 35g • sugars 23g • fibre 1g • protein 12g •
salt 0.2g

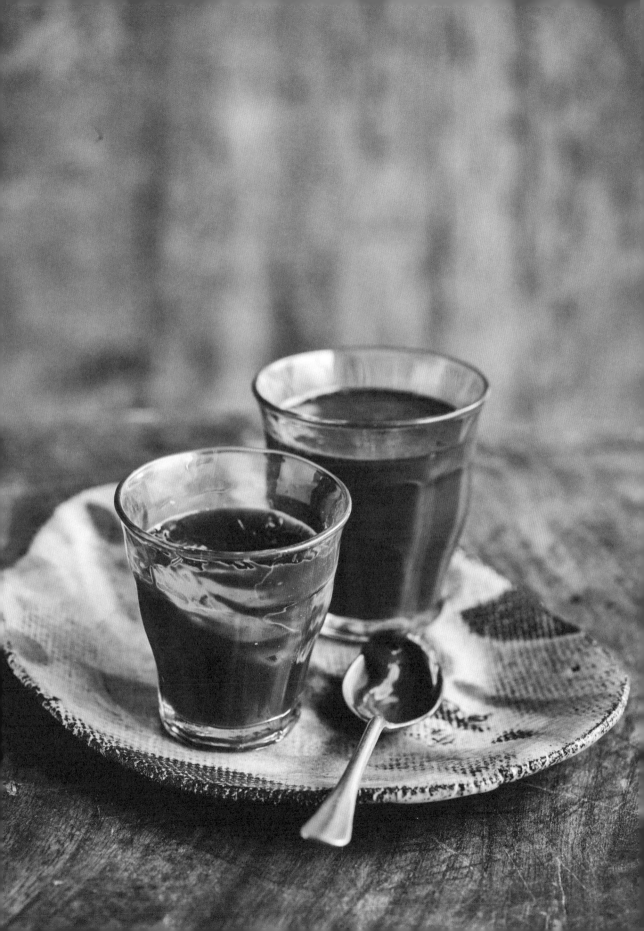

Sticky Cinnamon Figs

This makes a speedy dessert, which is special enough for entertaining friends. The cinnamon adds depth to the dish and is said to help moderate blood sugar levels.

🕐 Takes 10 mins   🥧 Serves 4

- 8 ripe fresh figs
- large knob of butter
- 2 tbsp maple syrup
- handful shelled pistachio nuts or flaked almonds
- ¼ tsp ground cinnamon
- live bio yogurt, to serve

1 Heat oven to 220C/200C fan/gas 7. Cut a deep cross in the top of each fig then ease the top apart like a flower. Sit the figs in a shallow baking dish and drop a small piece of the butter into the centre of each fruit. Drizzle the syrup over the figs, then sprinkle with the nuts and spice.

2 Bake for 5 mins until the figs are softened and the syrup and butter make a sticky sauce in the bottom of the dish. Serve warm, with the yogurt if you like.

BENEFITS vegetarian • 1 of 5 a day • gluten free
PER SERVING 137 kcals • fat 5g • saturates 1g • carbs 20g • sugars 19g • fibre 3g • protein 2g • salt 0.2g

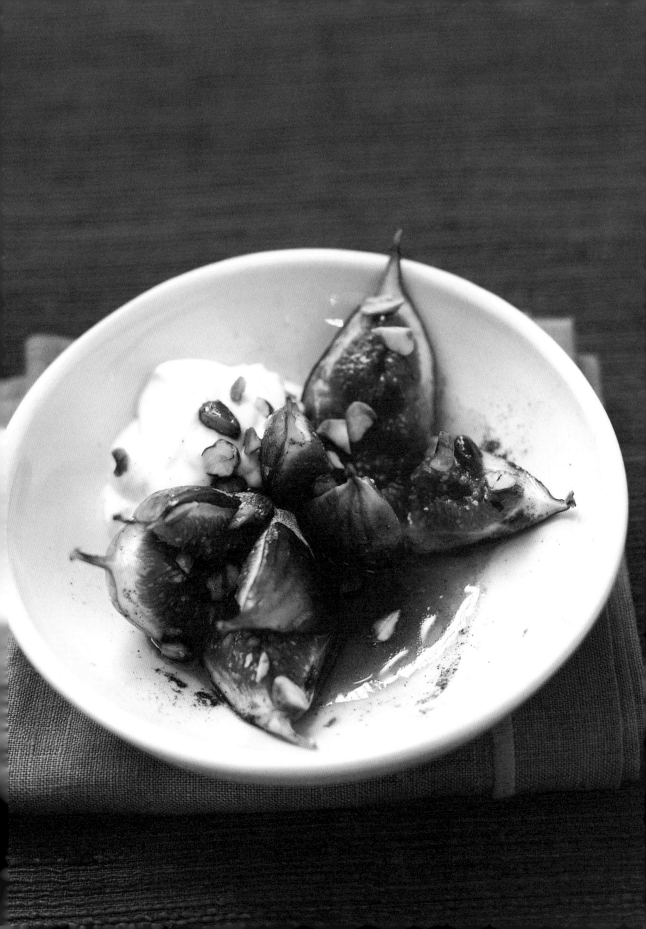

Oeufs au Lait

These little French vanilla custard puddings are deliciously creamy and surprisingly low in fat. They will keep in the fridge for up to 2 days.

🕐 Takes 40 minutes, plus chilling   🥧 Serves 4

- butter, for greasing
- 425ml/¾ pint milk
- 2 tbsp maple syrup
- 1 tsp vanilla extract
- 2 eggs

1 Butter 4 ramekins, about 150ml/¼ pint each. Heat oven to 160C/140C fan/gas 3. Have a roasting tin ready and put the kettle on. Pour the milk into a pan with the syrup and vanilla. Bring gently to the boil. Remove from the heat and cool for a few mins.

2 In a large bowl, beat the eggs until frothy. Slowly whisk in the milk. Set the ramekins in the roasting tin and divide the custard among them. Pour hot water around the ramekins to come halfway up the sides. Bake for 20 mins until just set, then cool and chill before serving.

BENEFITS vegetarian • gluten free
PER SERVING 134 kcals • fat 7g • saturates 3g • carbs 11g • sugars 11g • fibre 0g • protein 7g • salt 0.2g

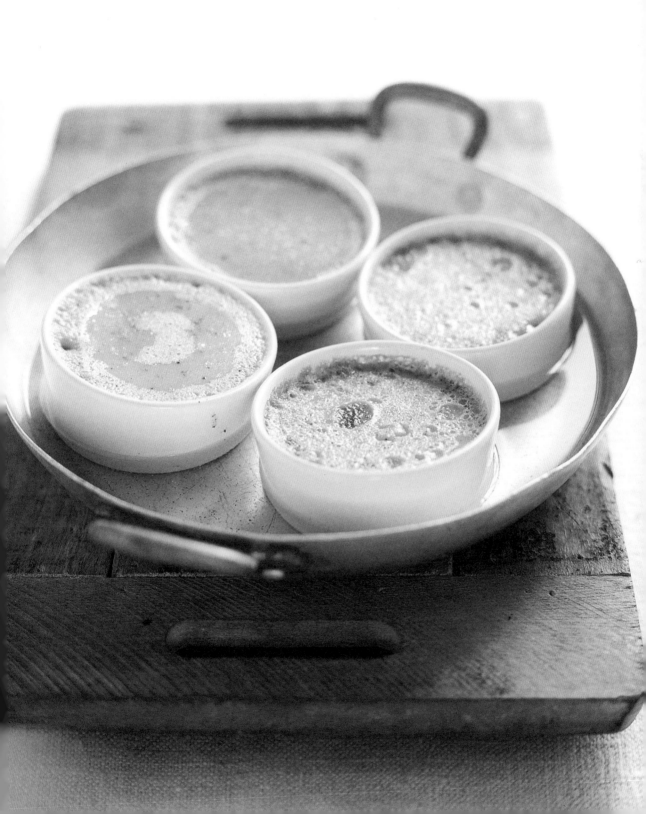

Vanilla Jellies with Apricot & Raspberry Compote

Jelly makes a deliciously light end to a meal. Our vanilla jellies have all the nourishing goodness of whole milk combined with the zesty flavours of fresh fruits.

🕐 Takes 30 mins, plus 3 hours chilling   ◑ Serves 4

- 4 sheets leaf gelatine
- 600ml/1 pint milk
- 3 tbsp maple syrup
- 2 tsp vanilla extract

FOR THE COMPOTE
- 500g/1lb 2oz apricots
- 3 tbsp apple juice
- 100g/4oz raspberries

1 Soak the gelatine for 10 mins in enough cold water to cover the leaves. Bring the milk and 1 tbsp syrup slowly to the boil. Remove from the heat and stir in the vanilla. Remove the gelatine from the soaking water, squeeze out the water, then stir into the milk until it has dissolved. Pour the jellies into 4 x 150ml/5fl oz moulds, cups or ramekins. Cool, then chill until set for about 3 hours.

2 Halve and stone the apricots, then cut each half into 4. Put in a pan with the apple juice and remaining syrup, then bring to a simmer. Gently cook for about 5 mins until the apricots are tender, but not pulpy. Remove from the heat, stir in the raspberries, then leave to cool.

3 Turn the jellies out onto 4 plates, then spoon compote around the edge.

BENEFITS vegetarian • low fat • 2 of 5 a day • gluten free
PER SERVING 203 kcals • fat 6g • saturates 3g • carbs 27g • sugars 26g • fibre 4g • protein 8g • salt 0.2g

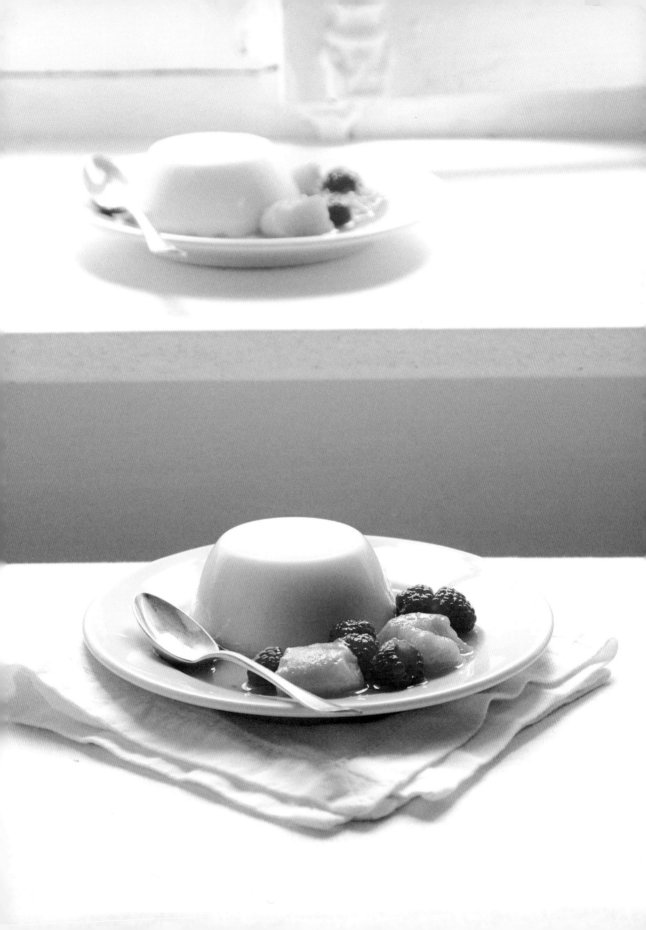

Pink Grapefruit, Raspberry & Mint Jellies

Forget sugary packaged jellies, these are fresh and tangy and so simple and quick to make for a sophisticated and elegant finish to any meal.

🕐 Takes 20 minutes, plus chilling ◔ Makes 6 jellies

- 5 sheets leaf gelatine
- 15g/½oz mint leaves, roughly chopped
- 1 pink grapefruit
- 100g/4oz small raspberries
- 2 ripe peaches, peeled, stoned and chopped

1 Soak the gelatine in a bowl of cold water for 10 mins. Boil 1 litre/1¾ pints water in the kettle and pour it over the mint leaves. Leave the mint to infuse for 5 minutes, then strain the liquid into a large jug. Squeeze the excess moisture from the soaked gelatine, then stir the gelatine into the hot mint mixture until dissolved. Set aside to cool.

2 Cut the peel and pith from the grapefruit with a sharp knife, then cut between the segments to release them, reserving any juice. Cut the segments into about 3 pieces each, then distribute the grapefruit, raspberries and peaches among 6 glasses. Stir the reserved grapefruit juice into the cooled mint jelly, then pour the jelly into the glasses and chill until set.

BENEFITS vegetarian • low fat • vit C • 1 of 5 a day • gluten free
PER JELLY 33 kcals • fat 0g • saturates 0g • carbs 5g • sugars 2g • fibre 2g • protein 2g • salt 0g

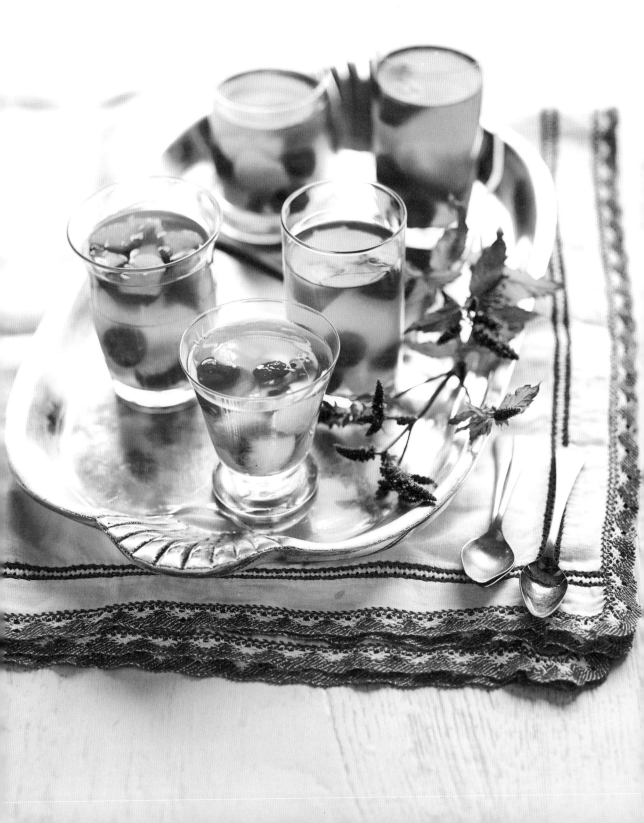

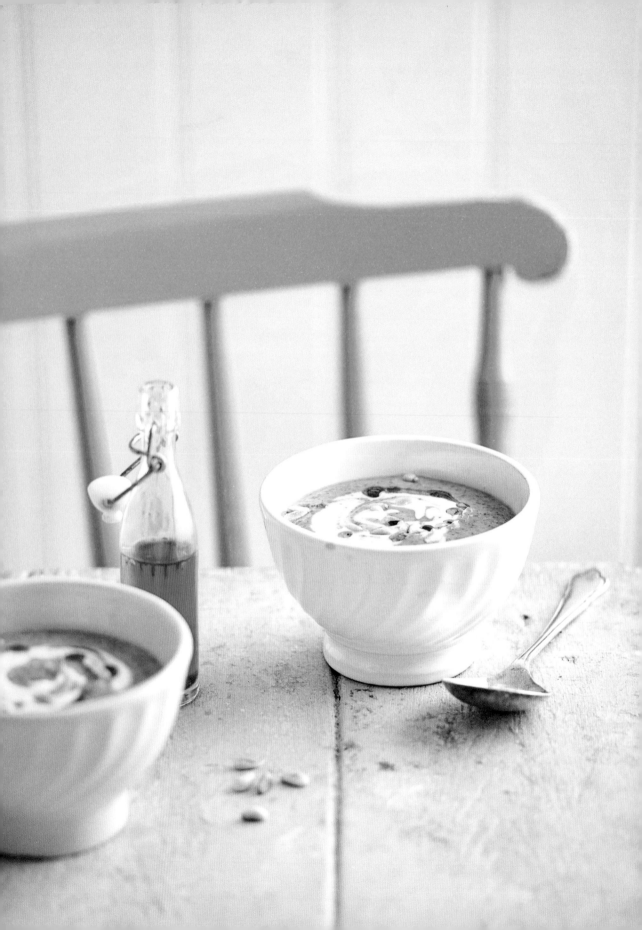

Your personal diet plans

· ·

Once you've followed our plans, here is your opportunity to create your own with the help of these blank charts. Choose from within each chapter to reap the benefits stipulated in the individual plans or for general healthy eating, pick recipes from anywhere in the book.

To make sure that you get the balance right for a whole day, select a breakfast, lunch and dinner, then add up all of the PER SERVING figures at the bottom of each recipe to make sure they don't exceed the daily figures (see below) based on what an average adult should consume each day.

Energy (Kilocalories): 2,000
Protein: 50g
Carbohydrate: 260g
Sugar: 90g
Fat: 70g
Saturated fat: 20g
Salt: 6g

	BREAKFAST	LUNCH	DINNER
Sunday			
Monday			
Tuesday			
Wednesday			
Thursday			
Friday			
Saturday			

	BREAKFAST	LUNCH	DINNER
Sunday			
Monday			
Tuesday			
Wednesday			
Thursday			
Friday			
Saturday			

	BREAKFAST	LUNCH	DINNER
Sunday			
Monday			
Tuesday			
Wednesday			
Thursday			
Friday			
Saturday			

	BREAKFAST	LUNCH	DINNER
Sunday			
Monday			
Tuesday			
Wednesday			
Thursday			
Friday			
Saturday			

Index

BBC goodfood

GET OUR
AWARD-WINNING DIGITAL MAGAZINE

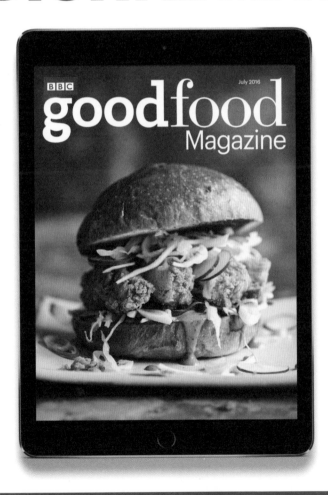

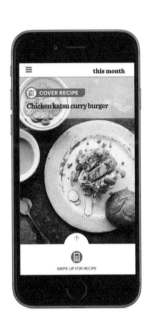

+ EASY-TO-VIEW RECIPE MODE

DOWNLOAD NOW

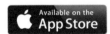
Available on the App Store